TRANSFORMATIVE
SHADOW
WORK

BOOKS BY LULU NICHOLSON

Codependency Recovery Workbook: Step-by-Step Guide to Overcome Fear of Abandonment, Stop People Pleasing, Set Boundaries, and Develop Healthy Relationships by Fostering Unconditional Self-Love

TRANSFORMATIVE
SHADOW
WORK

THE 3-PART SYSTEM TO EMBRACE YOUR HIDDEN SELF AND
TRANSCEND EMOTIONAL TRIGGERS & PAST TRAUMAS
TO REDUCE STRESS, ENHANCE PERSONAL GROWTH,
AND IMPROVE RELATIONSHIPS

LULU NICHOLSON

Contents

Navigating Inevitable Emotional

PART 2
DISCOVERING YOUR SHADOW SELF

Starting Your Trauma Recovery Journey

Integrating Your Shadow for a Whole You

PART 3
CELEBRATING PERSONAL GROWTH

06.

Enhancing Your Relationships Through Shadow Work

07.

Overcoming Common Shadow Work Challenges

08.

Celebrating Your Transformation

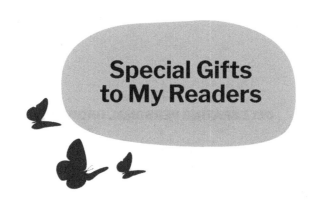

Special Gifts to My Readers

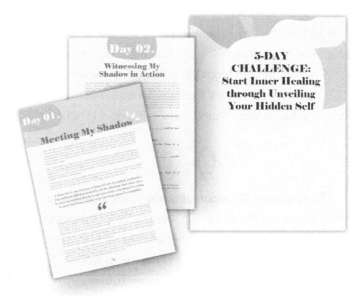

Included with your purchase of this book is the '**5-Day Challenge: Start Inner Healing Through Unveiling Your Hidden Self.**'

Simply scan the QR code or click the link below and provide the email address you'd like it delivered to. This 5-day program will help you begin your self-improvement journey on the right foot:

Day 1: MEETING MY SHADOW
Day 2: WITNESSING MY SHADOW IN ACTION
Day 3: INTEGRATING MY SHADOW
Day 4: ACCEPTING MY SHADOW
Day 5: BECOMING WHOLE

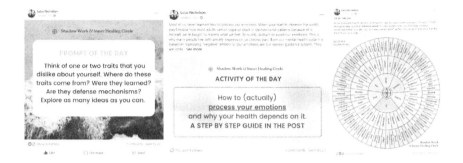

Additionally, I invite you to join the
'Shadow Work & Inner Healing Circle' Facebook Group
for Daily Prompts and Activities.

This new community is designed for beginners and those well into their journey, and it is suitable for:

- Anyone seeking to incorporate inner work into their daily routine and make it a lifelong practice.
- Anyone in search of support and accountability within a private, safe space.
- Anyone looking to connect with like-minded individuals.
- Anyone seeking tangible, practical steps and healing tools to delve deeper into their journey.
- Anyone (and I mean anyone) seeking to create change in their life!

To my loving husband and daughter,
who teach me so much about myself
and support me every step of the way.

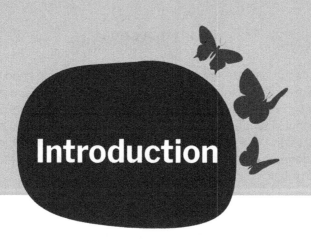

Introduction

We're afraid that if we fully surrender to our darkness, we'll never come back from it. We're afraid that if we show these ugly, unpalatable parts of ourselves, it will be too much for others; that nobody will love and accept us, and we'll be left alone with only the worst parts of ourselves for company. –Evanna Lynch

66

A Picture-Perfect Life—Or Is It?

We live in a time of filters and Photoshop, where everything isn't always as it seems. The rise of social media and influencer culture has made us aspire to live picture-perfect lives, or at least pretend to be.

Whether you are active on social media or not, you cannot deny the pressure that society places on you to succeed, accumulate wealth, achieve the perfect work-life balance, have a thriving social life, and still find time for practicing pilates and meditation.

A recurring thought you might have is that nothing you do is ever enough. No matter how much effort you make to obtain this "picture-perfect life," you always come up short. When comparing yourself to others, you realize that you aren't the smartest, slimmest, or most social person in the room. Suddenly, you become the problem, the imposter, the man or woman who is going nowhere, slowly.

In your desperate attempt to find reasons for not being good enough, it doesn't occur to you that perhaps this picture-perfect life you are striving for is just an illusion that corporations make trillions of dollars promoting. The perfect student, parent, and couple only exist on TV, Instagram, and magazines. In the real world, ordinary people are hustling their way up the corporate ladder, fighting personal demons, and doing their best to maintain relationships with others.

Like many others who have bought into the illusion of a picture-perfect life, you have been tricked into despising the very essence of what makes you authentic. Out of fear of public embarrassment, you hide unresolved trauma, emotional baggage, insecurities, and real-life challenges you are facing. What you don't realize is that these hidden aspects of your life are normal, natural, and common experiences that millions of people are dealing with.

The objective of this book is to challenge your belief of not feeling good enough and reintroduce you to your authentic self. Through exploring a new age concept and self-healing therapy called shadow work, you will be taken on a journey of rediscovering who you are and piecing together the beautiful story of your life.

Why Shadow Work?

Despite your best efforts, your life doesn't always go as planned. When you least expect it, factors outside of your control hijack your plans and cause delays or complete halts to your progress. However, this doesn't mean that you don't have a role to play in your suffering. If you take an honest assessment of your life, you can admit that certain toxic beliefs, emotional triggers, and self-sabotaging behaviors do more harm than good when seeking to improve the quality of your life.

There have been moments when you have lost control of your emotions and descended into what felt like hell. All you remember about the situation is feeling triggered, but the rest is a blur. When your emotions stabilize, and you return to a normal state, you wonder how such an insignificant event could have led to a hysterical reaction.

Reconciling the "acceptable" aspects of your identity with the dark aspects of your identity can feel like solving a murder mystery. You go back and forth trying to understand the connection between your thoughts, emotions, and behaviors. The math doesn't seem to add up because how you respond in your conscious state is completely different from when you are reacting unconsciously. You may not realize that your subconscious mind stores another part of your identity, your shadow self, which has not yet been fully integrated into who you are. It is what many people refer to as the dark side, or alter ego, that consists of parts of yourself that you repress or hide from others.

Shadow work is a therapeutic technique that works with your subconscious mind to introduce you to, and embrace, your shadow self. You can think of it as another side of your personality that contains qualities or behaviors you deem undesirable. Unresolved past trauma and emotional issues that have built up over the years also form part of your shadow. The goal of shadow work is to accept parts of your life story that you have hidden from yourself and others and heal from patterns of negative thinking and self-destructive habits. By coming face-to-face with the horrors of your past and embracing your life for what it is, you can develop a healthy self-concept and learn to be content with who you are.

The Value of Reading This Book

The ideal reader of this book isn't someone who believes their life is perfect but, instead, someone who is willing to admit that they are not satisfied with their current life situation.

You may be experiencing chronic stress and anxiety due to wearing many hats and trying your best not to disappoint others. You may be experiencing relationship problems as a result of emotional baggage from past relationships. You could also be at a stage of wanting to discover who you are but get caught in the middle between your real self and self-image.

To chip away at the false self-image, we will look at some of the mental and emotional issues that are blocking your personal growth, such as doubts, insecurities, fears, triggers, and low self-worth. Then, we will seek to address these issues using shadow work techniques like journaling, mindfulness meditation, cultivating self-compassion, and shadow integration.

For an enhanced reading experience, the book is divided into three sections:

- Part 1: Understanding Shadow Work (Chapters 1–3)

- Part 2: Discovering Your Shadow Self (Chapters 4–5)

- Part 3: Celebrating Personal Growth (Chapters 6–8)

The three-part system includes concrete examples and beginner-friendly exercises to make shadow work easy to incorporate into your everyday life. The system has been carefully designed to walk you through the shadow work process so you can gain the necessary skills to master each phase on your own. If this is your first time reading this book or using the shadow work process, it is recommended to go through the sections and read the chapters in order. In the second and third reading of the book, you can choose which sections or chapters you would like to focus on.

This book is a product of love written and published by a therapist-endorsed author and a life coach who is dedicated to the field of self-improvement, with a strong focus on psychology enriched with holistic principles and spiritual insights. My passion lies in guiding individuals on their path to self-discovery through my writings. I craft content centered around mental health, relationships, personal growth, and stress management. My approach blends evidence-based principles with practical exercises and relatable examples, aiming to make complex concepts accessible to my readers.

Having embarked on my transformative journey from a challenging past to a fulfilling present, I aim to write from a place of authenticity and share insights that I have learned through my exploration of consciousness and some amazing spiritual experiences I have had along the way. Although the internet is full of resources related to this subject, few delve deeply into the nature of the shadow self and shadow work as a practice. This is why I have decided to write this comprehensive book that compiles all of the necessary steps and skills to start your shadow work practice in the comfort of your home.

The purpose of this book is not to change you but rather to help you become more accepting and comfortable with who you are. Reading this book will open your eyes and broaden your perspective about the "self." You will be challenged to redefine who you are based on traits, strengths, values, and passions you discover about yourself along the way.

Trigger Warning

Some of the content included in this book may be triggering to sensitive readers. If you are living with a diagnosed mental health condition (or suspect that you may be living with an undiagnosed mental health condition), please consult a therapist before embarking on this journey. The information included in this book is not a substitute for seeking professional medical support.

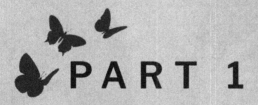

PART 1

UNDERSTANDING SHADOW WORK

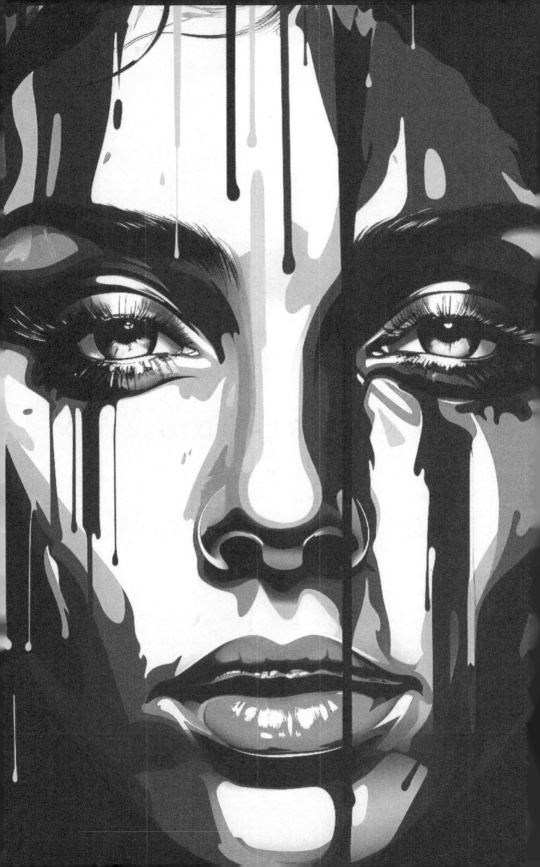

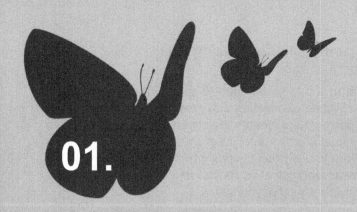

01.

Unveiling the Shadow Self

The shadow is needed now more than ever. We heal the world when we heal ourselves, and hope shines brightest when it illuminates the dark.
–Sasha Graham

Defining Shadow Work

Have you ever felt uneasy about being followed by a strange dark figure that never leaves your side? The shadow is the inanimate imposter that stalks you on a bright sunny day and is formed whenever you or an object blocks direct sunlight. Your shadow follows you and imitates your movements until the clouds move in and cover the beaming sun rays.

In psychology, the shadow is a metaphoric concept that is used to describe a hidden aspect of who you are, known as the shadow self. It is a dark and mysterious figure that gets exposed when you are emotionally triggered, then goes back into hiding when the trigger subsides. Just as abruptly as the shadow appears, it disappears without notice, leaving behind a trace of its existence in the form of emotional outbursts, self-destructive behaviors, alcohol and food binges, and anything else you might label as "taboo."

Shadow work is both a psychotherapeutic and spiritual practice that focuses on acknowledging, connecting, and integrating your shadow self with other known parts of your identity. Psychoanalyst Carl Jung is often credited for conceptualizing the practice of shadow work and giving us a practical framework to use when tapping into this hidden identity. The framework involves accepting that you have a dark side and taking steps to learn more about this aspect of yourself.

The goal of shadow work is not to judge or change who you are but rather to gain a richer and more balanced perspective of yourself. Don't be fooled by what you see or hear on social media—there is no such thing as a perfect life or perfect human being. We are all strong and broken in different ways, which enables us to live diverse and interesting lives that are shaped by unique life circumstances. At the heart of shadow work is the cultivation of self-awareness, which ultimately leads to greater self-acceptance and self-compassion.

Embracing your dark side is an empowering step to reclaiming lost dimensions of your personality so you can begin to see yourself as a whole person rather than a "good" or "bad" person. Carl Jung believed that the shadow self had the potential for creativity and building positive relationships, but only when it was understood and assimilated into your holistic identity.

The core focus of shadow work is to tap into your subconscious mind and unveil negative impulses, beliefs, memories, and habits that have been unconsciously influencing your behaviors and outlook on the world. While it is enough to simply acknowledge that you have these attributes pulling strings in the background, you can go a step further and seek to address and manage them. By doing the latter, you can effectively transform your thoughts and behavioral patterns and gain more control over your triggers and everyday reactions.

Shadow work is an empowering practice for everybody because we can all benefit from being more self-aware and self-actualized. Whether we choose to admit it or not, we possess a dark side that may be different from how we desire to perceive ourselves. For those of us who are not familiar with this dark side, the practice of shadow work can help us understand it better. Some people may find that their shadow carries trauma. This means that there may be some emotional scars from the past that have been left unaddressed. Shadow work can pull up these scars and assist in trauma recovery. It can also help trauma survivors accept and embrace their fears and become the best versions of themselves.

We need to be careful not to limit shadow work to resolving identity issues. On a broader level, shadow work can also help us confront our social and cultural conditioning, which impacts how we interact with others and the beliefs and prejudices we hold. Jung believed that the collective unconscious, which refers to the ideas, beliefs, and memories held by society as a whole, influences the personal shadow. In other words, the false and unkind messages spread in families, schools, workplaces, and the media can impact how individuals negatively perceive themselves and others. Thus, when addressing racism, corruption, disinformation, monopolization, violence, elitism, and environmental degradation as systemic issues, we refer to these as detrimental ideologies that influence the conduct of specific groups, shaping their interactions and relationships with one another.

The Benefits of Shadow Work

Shadow work improves the way you perceive yourself and your life. With heightened awareness, you have more options regarding what lifestyle you want to live, what types of relationships you want to cultivate, and what kind of future you aspire to. To give you a better understanding of how shadow work can enrich your life, here are some of the benefits you can look forward to:

- **self-awareness:** Shadow work teaches you how to recognize your thoughts and emotions, make the connection with your needs and wants, and learn how to meet them more healthily and build constructive habits.

- **clearer perception:** Self-knowledge, which is knowing who you are, allows you to see others and the world more clearly. Shadow work encourages you to look beyond the veil of your self-image and discover your authentic self, which brings about higher self-awareness. This enables you to sense how you are feeling or what you need internally and respond to the needs of your external environment.

- **pattern recognition:** Shadow work puts the truth in front of your eyes and reveals learned patterns that are holding you back. Since human beings are creatures of momentum and homeostasis, it is difficult to change patterns once they are formed. Nevertheless, shadow work encourages you to reflect on and consciously change how you think, feel, and behave toward experiences, which can break down this barrier and improve emotional well-being.

• **trigger identification:** As you learn to recognize patterns, you will be able to identify the source of your triggers in everyday situations. Shadow work enables you to look behind your emotional triggers and address the past trauma and pain that keeps resurfacing whenever you are feeling stressed, fearful, or vulnerable. By understanding your triggers, you can effectively manage them and prevent explosive reactions.

• **emotional healing:** Shadow work can assist in uncovering and confronting unresolved trauma, emotional baggage, and other psychological problems that interfere with your everyday functioning and capacity to connect with yourself and others.

• **generational trauma healing:** Shadow work helps you reconcile your past, form new thoughts and behavioral patterns, and reach a place of acceptance for who you are. This ensures that you heal and end the cycle of trauma that you inherited as a result of your parents' upbringing or the systemic ills of the community you grew up in.

• **enhanced energy and physical health:** Shadow work can alleviate emotional distress, which improves your overall mental and emotional well-being and lowers the risk of physical pain and diseases, as well as obsessive or addictive behaviors. Feeling calm and balanced inwardly radiates as high energy and positive moods outwardly.

• **personal growth and self-acceptance:** Shadow work can help you get out of your shell and explore new dimensions of your personality. You gain a deeper appreciation for who you are and the unique life path you are on. Shadow work can also help you accept that you are not perfect, nor are you expected to be. This can create a renewed commitment to live your life unapologetically!

• **healthy self-esteem and greater confidence:** Integrating your shadow with your conscious identity allows you to show up with greater confidence because there are no more secrets to hide. The self-doubt that you had hidden for many years or the physical attributes you struggled to accept about yourself become things you can accept. Not all of your shadow traits will be undesirable qualities, but when you come across some that are, you will lovingly acknowledge and address the deeper wounds so they don't get in the way of your progress.

• **increased compassion toward others:** Shadow work helps you manage your projection when interacting with others. How other people feel or behave is less likely to trigger you. As a result, you can generate feelings of compassion toward others because you are no longer resisting your dark side mirrored by them. Instead, you can see them as whole, separate individuals who likely have their hidden inner battles to face.

• **improved relationships:** Shadow work focuses on strengthening the relationship you have with yourself. It teaches you how to put yourself first, which means making self-care a priority and forming healthier habits. Only when your needs are met, and your metaphoric cup is full will you have more time, patience, and value to offer your loved ones and be able to build stronger bonds with them.

• **boosted creativity:** Shadow work uncovers repressed ideas, desires, and goals that are buried in your subconscious mind. You may have rejected these positive and creative aspects of yourself during a time when you were under severe stress and placed your survival as a priority. Now that you are in a better position to tap into your imagination and dream again, you can reconnect with your creative side.

• **hidden talent discovery:** You can use shadow work to discover the "gold in your shadow bags," which refers to your untapped or unknown strengths and resources. This "golden" aspect of your shadow is more significant than your dark side. However, due to being overshadowed by your traumas and emotional wounds, it hasn't gotten the opportunity to thrive. Shadow work reveals and gives attention to this side of yourself so you can become more than what you dreamed of.

• **psychological integration and maturity:** Shadow work helps you develop a whole, stable, and integrated self. The process challenges the illusions that you have held about who you are and invites you to come face-to-face with the truth. You get the opportunity to see yourself and your life as it is, not as you desire it to be. As a result, you develop psychological maturity and learn how to face challenges like an adult.

How the Shadow Self Manifests in Daily Life

We all have basic human needs, like physiological needs of safety and security or psychological needs of affection and a sense of belonging. To feel secure as a child, these basic human needs must be met. If you were raised in an environment where some of your basic needs were threatened, a part of you may have felt unsafe. For instance, your parents' lack of consistent affection could have made you feel anxious. Or being rejected by your teachers or classmates could have threatened your sense of belonging. Situations like these set the foundation for the shadow self, the part of you that doesn't feel safe and accepted and overcompensates by changing aspects of itself to "fit in."

When you came into the world, you were open and free of judgment, but as you grew older, you had experiences that caused you to judge yourself. Starting in early childhood, you began disconnecting from parts of your identity that you considered "undesirable," such as showing anger or needing reassurance from others. This may have included disconnecting from the best parts of yourself, like your courage, generosity, and sensitivity.

Essentially, you cut away anything (good or bad) that you couldn't find a way to integrate into your personality. This is because, during childhood and adolescence, young children strive to become, in a sense, "normal," which causes them to adopt the behaviors of their social group. In so doing, you divorced yourself from anything that didn't get acceptance or approval from your environment, including your parents, relatives, teachers, friends, or society as a whole. Those unacceptable things about yourself were pushed into the shadow.

In reality, you didn't cut off parts of yourself. All of the traits and behaviors that were deemed undesirable within the first 20 years of your life were stored in your unconscious mind. Although you denied them to yourself and others, in an attempt to get rid of them, they didn't go anywhere. Instead, you repressed them. Suddenly, you became "two people." Your personality came to include the persona, which is the personality that you show to the public, representing all of the different social masks that you wear among various groups and situations, and the shadow self, which remains private or hidden. It most often appears when you are emotionally triggered or presented with situations that threaten your sense of safety.

The reason why your shadow self is hidden is that it feels dangerous, embarrassing, or inappropriate. It contradicts everything that you have come to love and accept about yourself, such as your easy-going, confident, and resilient nature. Hiding the shadow self is seen as a way of protecting your self-image, status, reputation, and personal brand. You have witnessed firsthand how cruel society can be to people whom they deem "weird," "weak," or "troubled," so you do your best to hide your pain, bad habits, and destructive behaviors from others.

Embracing one aspect of your identity while disowning the other creates internal confusion and conflict. Every once in a while, whenever your triggers are activated, you may find yourself acting out of character. The truth is that it isn't out of character but rather an expression of a side of yourself that you haven't acknowledged and accepted, which operates without your full awareness. When this other side emerges, your conscious mind goes to sleep, and another personality surfaces and takes control. This explains why you may sound, talk, or behave differently or see the world through a different lens. In this state, you do not possess the conscious awareness to reflect on your behaviors and notice that you are acting differently.

Moreover, the shadow can choose to appear through projections. Projection happens when you see things in others that you subconsciously recognize within yourself. Whatever qualities you deny in yourself are the qualities you judge harshly in others. Anything that is buried within you and considered inappropriate is projected onto others. This process doesn't happen consciously, meaning that you aren't aware of your projections. Your ego uses them as a psychological defense to prevent your shadow from surfacing. The ego would much rather have you believe that other people are wrong and you are right than doing the work to address your harmful behavioral patterns.

The shadow self is not necessarily destructive when it is embraced and managed appropriately. It is the lack of acknowledgment and acceptance that makes you feel out of control when your shadow manifests. As Jung explained, "A man who is unconscious of himself acts in a blind, instinctive way and is in addition fooled by all the illusions that arise when he sees everything that he is not conscious of in himself coming to meet him from outside as projections upon his neighbor" (Jeffrey, 2019).

The worst-kept secret is that everybody has a conscious and unconscious self. Even in cases where individuals do not have a history of trauma, there are aspects of their identity that are known and unknown. The fear of judgment is what prevents us from having open conversations about our shadows and the negative emotions, thoughts, and behaviors we are battling with.

Perfection is, therefore, a standard that human beings cannot realistically attain because of our dual nature. There will always be things about us that we know and accept, know and reject, or have not yet discovered.

Self-actualization, the process of becoming who you truly are, is the closest that you will get to perfection. The process involves examining the contrast and relationship between your conscious and unconscious selves and working toward integrating them and becoming whole. Undergoing this process helps you find meaning and purpose in your life and express an authentic identity.

The Impact of Unacknowledged Shadows

At this stage, you are familiar with the concept of the shadow self and the benefits of shadow work. However, there may still be a part of you that resists vulnerability and is open to this process. Even though you know that some issues from the past have held you back in certain areas of your life, you fear what might happen when you start exploring your subconscious mind.

The truth is that whether you choose to acknowledge and accept your shadow self or not, it will continue to appear and disappear in your life. The only difference when you decide to accept your shadow is that you gain control over your unconscious thoughts, emotions, and behaviors and can choose how to process and respond to them.

An unacknowledged shadow self can interfere with the order, stability, and harmony that you are working hard to build and maintain in your life. It appears and disappears spontaneously and manifests behaviors that can be considered destructive and unproductive. Moreover, when your unacknowledged shadow self does appear, you will have no control over your reactions because you don't fully understand what might have triggered you and what traumas have been brought to the surface.

Another fear that may be holding you back from committing to this process is being exposed to your dark side. For many years, you have accepted your conscious self as being your whole identity, not realizing that there is another side to you. Due to the shame of having to acknowledge personal weaknesses, you would rather pretend that your shadow self isn't relevant to your life.

Repressing your shadow self only causes it to become more powerful and destructive. It's like telling a child that they cannot eat the candy on the table. The more they focus on not grabbing a piece of candy, the stronger the temptation to eat it becomes. When your energy is focused on hiding your shadow, you may find it more challenging to control your unconscious thoughts, emotions, and behaviors. Your dark side will show up in unexpected ways to seek your attention. Some of the behaviors that manifest due to an unacknowledged shadow self include:

- unexplained anxiety or panic attacks
- exaggerated emotional outbursts to minor situations
- self-soothing with addictive substances like recreational drugs, prescription medicine, and alcohol
- ongoing conflict in your relationships that are sparked by minor inconveniences
- feeling increasingly vulnerable to stress and not being able to recover quickly
- engaging in negative self-talk and thinking the worst of others
- making impulsive decisions that get you in trouble or compromise your relationships
- self-sabotaging by engaging in risky behaviors that risk your safety or get you in trouble with the law

The choice to acknowledge your shadow or not boils down to the level of control you would like to have over your psychological state of mind. Do you want to be surprised by your shadow at unexpected times, or do you want to sense your shadow emerging and take preventative measures to ensure you stay in control of your thoughts, emotions, and behaviors?

Shadow Work Journaling

At the end of each chapter, you will be allowed to pause and reflect on your shadow work journey by completing some journal prompts. You may be familiar with the standard form of journaling, where you express your thoughts and feelings in a notebook. Shadow work journaling is similar, except the objective is to bring the shadow to your conscious awareness by exploring questions that allow you to dig deep into your mind.

The nature of the prompts challenges you to recall memories and events from the past or unpack your belief system or personal feelings toward yourself and others. The prompts are merely a guide to helping you travel further into your childhood or beyond your existing mental pathways. Answer the prompts as honestly as you can without thinking too hard about your responses.

Shadow Work Journal Prompts

1. In your opinion, what is your best personality trait?

2. In your opinion, what is your worst personality trait?

3. What strength makes you valuable at work?

4. When do you feel the happiest about yourself?

5. What role did friendships play in your childhood?

6. What childhood memories bring the most inner joy?

7. What childhood memories cause the most pain?

8. When was the last time you felt like a failure? What happened?

9. Who do you admire most in your life? Why?

**10. What relationships in your life have been
the toughest to manage? Why?**

**11. Have you ever experienced body image issues?
Describe your journey thus far.**

12. When do you feel doubtful about yourself?

13. What grudge are you still holding on to?

14. What behaviors irritate you the most in others?

15. What is your number one relationship pet peeve?

16. What are your biggest fears when it comes to being vulnerable?

17. How often have you received support in the past?

18. What is something that people don't know about you?

19. What do you envy in other people? Why?

20. Who owes you an apology? Why?

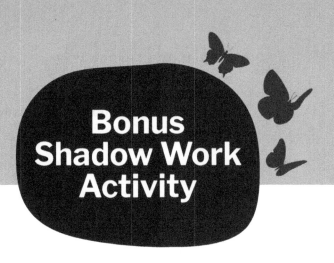

Bonus Shadow Work Activity

Which Shadow Archetypes Resonate with You the Most?

Learning about shadow archetypes can be a great way to personalize your shadow and study the characteristics that form part of your shadow self framework. This is a great starting point, especially when you are unaware of your shadow personality. Moreover, you may find it easier to identify and address certain thoughts, emotions, and behaviors manifesting from your shadow self when you are familiar with your dark personality.

In Jungian psychology, personalities are called archetypes. Jung identified four major archetypes: the persona, self, shadow, and anima/animus (Hill, 2023). Among the persona, self, and shadow, there are inner forces that are gendered, which describe our soul life, or the energies that operate on an unconscious level. These are known as the anima (feminine) and animus (masculine) (Farah, 2015). Unlike the real world, where your personality matches the gender you were born with, the soul assigns the opposite gender characteristics to men and women. Thus, the anima is a feminine energy in the male psyche, and the animus is a masculine energy in the female psyche. This creates a balance between the conscious and unconscious self, allowing men and women to possess dual energies.

According to Jung, the four main archetypes can be expressed in creative ways and manifest as 12 archetypical figures (Hill, 2023). The archetypes draw inspiration from prehistoric archetypes that have existed across multiple cultures and periods. Furthermore, archetypes describe the dual nature of identities. Each archetype has a conscious and unconscious side, which depicts the healed and unhealed version of yourself.

Go through the following 12 archetypes and their shadow equivalents, and examine which ones come close to describing your shadow self. Rate them by checking one of the following statements: fully agree, somewhat agree, not sure, somewhat disagree, fully disagree.

Make a note of the shadow archetypes that you fully agreed, somewhat agreed, and not sure with and refer back to them throughout the shadow work process to understand your shadow personality better.

The Ruler

The ruler is a goal-orientated, success-driven person who is either in a position of authority or aspires to have authority. They are natural-born leaders who perform well under pressure and gain respect from others. They rely on sound logic and strategy to make decisions instead of impulsive or emotional inclinations. They pride themselves in traditional values and have a peaceful home life and pleasant union with their partner or spouse.

Shadow self: The dark side of the ruler shows up when they are controlling others (especially when they feel insecure). Whenever they feel disrespected, misunderstood, or underappreciated, they may become angry and uncooperative. The ruler may also struggle to apologize, admit mistakes, and take accountability for their shortcomings out of fear of appearing weak, damaging their reputation, or undermining their authority.

Does this archetypal shadow impact the way you move in the world?
- fully agree
- somewhat agree
- not sure
- somewhat disagree
- fully disagree

The Caregiver

The caregiver is a nurturing person who derives a sense of purpose from helping others. They develop maturity early in their life and feel responsible for taking care of their friends and family. Their natural maternal instinct gives them a desire to have children, nurture animals, or volunteer at shelters. The caregiver is dedicated and passionate about improving the well-being of others.

Shadow self: The dark of the caregiver shows up when they start to feel taken for granted for supporting others. This may stem from a lack of proper boundaries and the ability to say no to others. They may also struggle to prioritize their needs, practice self-care, and advocate for what they want. This breeds resentment and low self-worth, which are often suppressed.

Does this archetypal shadow impact the way you move in the world?
- fully agree
- somewhat agree
- not sure
- somewhat disagree
- fully disagree

29

The Everyman

The everyman is a sociable and outgoing person who craves acceptance and a sense of belonging. They understand human behavior and are naturally people-magnets. Being part of a community and having strong connections is important to them because they offer stability and grounding. They prefer quality over quantity when it comes to relationships, so they would rather opt for a night spent indoors with family than a night spent partying with a group of friends.

Shadow self: The dark side of the everyman manifests when they feel alienated, rejected, or disconnected from other people. This can be a crushing experience that raises feelings of worthlessness and desperation. They may display people-pleasing tendencies like changing their behaviors to suit other people when they feel pressure to fit in or gain approval from others.

Does this archetypal shadow impact the way you move in the world?
- fully agree   • somewhat agree   • not sure
  • somewhat disagree   • fully disagree

The Creator

The creator is a highly imaginative and eccentric person who uses their mind, hands, voice, or natural-born talent to create something. They are hardworking risk-takers who are not satisfied with a mediocre life. Unlike the ruler, who is driven by success, the creator is driven by the ability to self-actualize and make a positive impact on the world. They often inspire others to freely express who they are and live an authentic and meaningful life.

Shadow self: The dark side of the creator manifests whenever they feel overwhelmed by the weight of their own creative mind. They might come up with innovative ideas but cannot execute and follow through until the end. Due to being non-conformists, they may abandon social norms and ethics in support of their ideologies. Thus, creators can struggle to maintain healthy relationships, achieve financial stability, and embrace adult responsibilities.

Does this archetypal shadow impact the way you move in the world?
- fully agree   • somewhat agree   • not sure
  • somewhat disagree   • fully disagree

The Innocent

The innocent is a person who is unapologetically themselves. They have a childlike spirit that comes across as playful and innocent. An adult with this personality has a romantic and uncorrupted view of the world. Like an innocent child, they are hopeful, forgiving, and optimistic. They make decisions based on how they intuitively feel or know to be true about their life. The innocent individual thrives in harmonious environments and relationships and can feel disorientated by chaos and unexpected life events.

Shadow self: The dark side of the innocent manifests as being overly dependent on others for survival. They might struggle with adult life's pressures and demands, forcing them to mature and stand on their own. The innocent individual can also display naivety, particularly when trusting the wrong people. Due to their idealistic and empathetic nature, they choose to see people through their own filters rather than accepting people for who they show themselves to be.

Does this archetypal shadow impact the way you move in the world?
· fully agree   · somewhat agree   · not sure
· somewhat disagree   · fully disagree

The Explorer

The explorer is a curious, adventure-seeking person who is passionate about learning, making discoveries, and bettering themselves. The explorer's unquenchable zest for knowledge makes their life interesting and constantly evolving. They are happiest when they are problem-solving, building skills, or conquering a challenge. Due to their openness to experiences, the explorer may have unconventional ideas and beliefs about life, which pushes them away from tradition and social norms.

Shadow self: The dark side of the explorer is being plagued by fear of stepping outside their comfort zone. Internally, they may feel a longing to question or challenge ideas but decide that it is safer to conform to the rules and follow social norms. As a result, they feel angry for not having the courage to pursue knowledge and live as they wish. This may lead to living a double life, developing addictions, and performing risky behaviors when under the influence of mind-numbing substances.

Does this archetypal shadow impact the way you move in the world?
· fully agree   · somewhat agree   · not sure
· somewhat disagree   · fully disagree

The Warrior

The warrior is a courageous person who goes after what they want despite being afraid. They have a positive attitude that enables them to endure hardships and stay committed to their goals. Part of what makes a warrior mentally strong is their high level of self-awareness. They embrace both strengths and weaknesses and tackle emotional issues head-on.

Shadow self: The dark side of the warrior shows up when they stubbornly fight for causes or goals that do not serve them, simply to prove a point to their friends or family. This may stem from being dismissed or criticized as a child by parents or school teachers. The result is feeling like they are not good enough and using goals or big dreams to gain validation from others.

Does this archetypal shadow impact the way you move in the world?
- fully agree   - somewhat agree   - not sure
- somewhat disagree   - fully disagree

The Outlaw

The outlaw is a radical thinker who prides themselves in not conforming to social norms. They are curious about the world and willing to test assumptions, even if it means denouncing what most people believe is right. The outlaw is passionate about using their position and personal power to make a positive impact in society and fight injustice. They may be an activist, conspiracy theorist, or controversial social commentator who is determined to expose the elite's agendas and bring about social change.

Shadow self: The shadow of the outlaw is similar to the shadow of the explorer, except for the fact that when given power, the unhealed outlaw can be reckless, make irrational decisions, and act in ways that do not serve the interests of the masses (even if that is the intention). They might also be controversial for the sake of being controversial instead of seeking truth and presenting practical solutions.

Does this archetypal shadow impact the way you move in the world?
- fully agree   - somewhat agree   - not sure
- somewhat disagree   - fully disagree

The Magician

The magician is a sensitive and intuitive person who is aware of their unconscious thoughts, emotions, and behaviors and uses them as tools for personal development. You can think of the magician as the mature version of the innocent, who displays more self-awareness and self-regulation. They are quiet, introverted, and live isolated from others, which sometimes makes them appear as cold, detached, and unfriendly.

Shadow self: The dark side of the magician manifests when their strengths also become their weaknesses. For instance, their sensitive nature might cause them to absorb the feelings of others to the extent of being emotionally drained. Their highly intuitive nature can cause them to overanalyze experiences, become paranoid, and struggle to differentiate between perception and reality.

Does this archetypal shadow impact the way you move in the world?
- fully agree   • somewhat agree   • not sure
        • somewhat disagree   • fully disagree

The Lover

The lover is a sensual and lighthearted person who enjoys the finer things in life. They are trusting and welcoming of others and enjoy the process of forming new relationships. The lover tends to get attention even when they are not asking for it because of how comfortable they are in their skin and how attuned they are to their needs. They feel happiest when engaging in creative, social, and sensory experiences that make them feel good.

Shadow self: The dark side of the lover shows up when they suppress their emotions and avoid showing vulnerability. This may stem from being hurt by past relationships and developing trust issues and other insecurities. It can also stem from being raised by avoidant or dismissive parents who didn't show affection or validate their child's needs. As adults, they struggle to love and accept themselves or receive love from others. This can lead to promiscuity, depression, and obsessive behaviors.

Does this archetypal shadow impact the way you move in the world?
- fully agree   • somewhat agree   • not sure
        • somewhat disagree   • fully disagree

The Jester

The jester is a bubbly and easy-going person who enjoys making others feel good about themselves. They tend to use humor to make others laugh and lighten the mood. As a leader, the jester is friendly and approachable, which makes them admired by their followers. They gain people's trust by not taking life too seriously and being a hopeful optimist.

Shadow self: The dark side of the jester manifests as ignorance of the rough realities of life. This might lead to irresponsible decisions, impulsive behaviors, and the manipulation of others. The jester may turn to addictive behaviors or obsessions to numb their emotional distress and avoid facing reality. They struggle to address real-life issues and confront challenges head-on, which creates a cycle of hiding and numbing pain.

Does this archetypal shadow impact the way you move in the world?
- fully agree   • somewhat agree   • not sure
- somewhat disagree   • fully disagree

The Sage

The sage has a similar personality to the magician, except the sage is the source of wisdom, whereas the magician strives to manifest wisdom. Thus, the sage can be seen as the mature version of the magician, who is balanced, emotionally regulated, and self-actualized. The sage seeks order and mental clarity. They prefer to see things for how they truly are rather than buy into illusions. The individual may also possess spiritual inclinations that make them effective in healing and counseling others.

Shadow self: The dark side of the sage manifests when their search for order and harmony causes them not to take any actions. They become preoccupied with observing reality and experiences instead of participating in them. The sage can also develop moral superiority because of what they have discovered about themselves, which creates a disconnect from other people. They might struggle to empathize or relate with others or enjoy the small joys that life has to offer.

Does this archetypal shadow impact the way you move in the world?
- fully agree   • somewhat agree   • not sure
- somewhat disagree   • fully disagree

Shadow work is a therapeutic process that can help you integrate your conscious and unconscious self, cultivating a whole and authentic identity. In the following chapter, we will take a closer look at the shadow work process and the steps you will need to embark on.

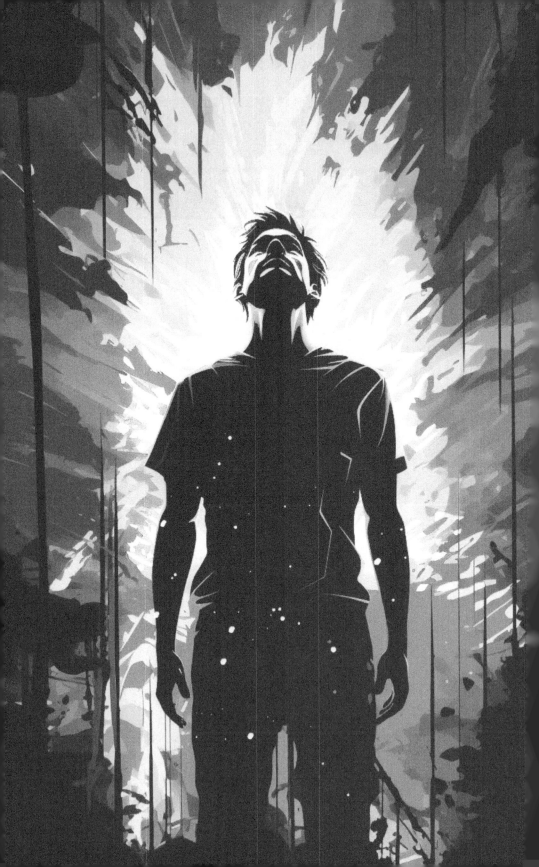

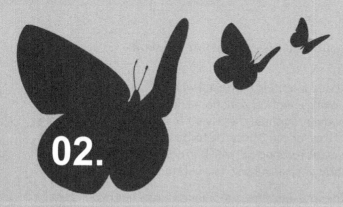

02.

How Do You Practice Shadow Work

Our shadows hold the essence of who we are. They hold our most treasured gifts. By facing these aspects of ourselves, we become free to experience our glorious totality: the good and the bad, the dark and the light. –Debbie Ford

Understanding the Shadow Work Process

An essential element when preparing for shadow work is understanding the basic process. This will help you manage your expectations and go into it feeling confident in your ability to follow through until the end. The basic process is flexible, meaning that you can decide how deeply to practice each step and what exercises to include or exclude. The process can be summarized in the following four steps:

Step 1: Identify Your Shadow

An important and ongoing part of shadow work is identifying your shadow self whenever it emerges. Ideally, the aim is to pick up on the warning signs of emotional triggers and respond decisively. However, for beginners, this can be a challenging task. For now, you are only expected to recognize your shadow regardless of when it shows up (i.e., before or after triggers).

Get into the habit of documenting moments when your unconscious self emerges and the specific events or situations that trigger it. For example, by tracking your moods throughout the day, you can pick up on significant mood disturbances that occur. These disturbances could be once-off, such as when you receive a phone call with bad news. Or the disturbances could happen regularly, such as having a weekly meeting with your boss.

Making a note of these experiences in a journal can help you identify your shadow self and connect real-life experiences with manifestations of your triggers and traumas. Moreover, be curious about the situations in your life that evoke your unconscious self; these could be situations connected to past traumas, failures, or destructive behaviors you are engaging in.

Step 2: Intuitive Drawing

Drawing can be a great way to mentally picture and connect with your shadow. If you are a visual learner, the aid of a drawing can help you make your unconscious self feel more real and tangible. You don't need to be a talented artist to practice intuitive drawing since you will not be graded on your artwork. The main idea is to creatively express your dark side as you sense it without thinking too hard about what you are drawing on paper.

This exercise is guided by your intuition, which means that your choice of craft materials, the object that you draw, the colors you use, and the time that it takes to complete your drawing are decided by your intuition. Your job is to go with the flow and avoid editing your drawing or structuring the creative process.

After you have completed the drawing, analyze your artwork and interpret its symbolic meaning. For example, if your shadow drawing filled the entire piece of paper, that could be symbolic of how intensely it is making its presence felt inside. If the drawing is in dark and dull colors, that might symbolize the negative and destructive thoughts or emotions you are feeling; however, if some vibrant colors are used, perhaps your shadow is feeling creative and playful.

You can also analyze the object you draw and what that symbolizes. For instance, your shadow might be depicted as a specific animal or insect with traits that are similar to how you are feeling. Alternatively, it could be depicted as an abstract shape that has a metaphoric meaning. There is a lot of information that you can extract from your drawing to gain insight into how your shadow self chooses to express itself at this present moment.

Step 3: Dialogue With Your Shadow

The previous step encourages you to connect with your shadow self. However, once you have made the connection, the following step is to engage with this aspect of yourself by starting a dialogue. You can decide whether to interpret this step literally or figuratively. For example, it might help you to imagine that you are talking to a younger version of yourself, the little child, teenager, or young adult who survived a painful season in your life.

Alternatively, you can engage with your shadow through self-reflection practices like journaling, meditation, and visualization. These methods help you tap into your subconscious mind and explore dimensions of your unconscious self as though you were getting to know someone for the first time. For these self-reflection practices to be successful, go into the process with an open mind, a nonjudgmental attitude, and the readiness to be surprised by what you discover.

Dialoguing with your shadow can evoke unpleasant memories and emotions. This is intentional and part of the healing process. Your greatest challenge will be to learn how to acknowledge and accept what you are shown or what you discover without judging or shaming yourself or over-identifying with any particular experience. For example, you should be able to replay a painful scene from childhood and empathize with the little child who went through the experience; however, reminding yourself at the same time that you are no longer the little child reliving the trauma—you are the adult who is no longer in that vulnerable position.

To gain rich insights from dialoguing with your shadow, practice going into the process with a sense of curiosity, seeking answers and being open to receiving suggestions or revelations. A useful tip is to have a few open-ended questions that you take into your shadow work sessions. If you are journaling, these questions could serve as your journal prompts. If you are meditating or speaking directly to a younger version of yourself, pose the questions into the atmosphere and patiently wait for intuitive responses.

The responses can arise as an audible voice, mental words or pictures, bodily sensations, or synchronicities (i.e. symbolic coincidences). The particular method that the shadow uses to communicate back to you depends on what you can easily discern and understand. For instance, if you are somebody who isn't aware of synchronicities, this won't be how your shadow communicates with you.

Step 4: Uncover the Shadow's Agenda

The shadow can cause chaos, but it is certainly not there to make your life miserable. The shadow manifests for a specific purpose or motivation, to help you in some way. Consider the motivation for smoking a cigarette. While the habit is destructive, the intention behind it is good. The smoker picks up a cigarette because they desire to unwind and relieve tension. This motivation sustains the behavior until it becomes an addictive habit that they have very little control over.

The final step in the shadow work process is to learn why your shadow appears in certain situations and motivates you to react negatively. What is its agenda? Think deeply about what benefits come with choosing destructive behaviors. There is something that you unconsciously gain from reacting to situations in what might seem unhealthy ways. If there wasn't anything to gain, you wouldn't be motivated to react in that manner when triggered.

Since the shadow self is born from pain and insecurity, the purpose or motivations behind the manifestations of your shadow are related to trauma-based coping mechanisms. In other words, the reason why you choose certain behaviors is because they feel safe, reliable, and protective. They help you cope with stress and anxiety in a manner that feels familiar. If you were to trace your coping mechanisms, you would find a trail leading back to early childhood. The behaviors that made you feel safe and protected then might be the behaviors that you rely on to feel safe and protected as an adult.

Uncovering the shadow's agenda won't make your shadow disappear for good. However, it can help you pull unconscious behaviors into your conscious reality and have more control over your actions. Using the analogy of the smoker, once they understand their motivation for smoking a cigarette, they have more choices when it comes to choosing how to address their anxious feelings.

Best Practices for Shadow Work

The shadow work process will only work if you work it. There are different ways that you can enhance your healing journey and ensure you get as much value out of it as possible. Next are beginner-friendly practices that you can incorporate into your daily life. These practices can be used to examine your thoughts, analyze your interactions with others, and reflect on your behaviors.

Look for Recurring Themes

When examining your thoughts, emotions, or behaviors, determine whether you reinforce a theme. A theme is a universal idea or message that forms the basis of a storyline. Due to past experiences, there could be core themes that you have adopted which influence your outlook and perceptions. For example, if you have a history of being neglected by others, a core theme in your life could be abandonment. Thus, whenever you feel as though people in your life are pulling away from you, the thought of being abandoned is triggered.

Here are some questions to help you find recurring themes:

- What intense emotions are triggered regularly?

- What behaviors in others do you find difficult to tolerate?

- What pushes your buttons about your partner?

- What do you react negatively to at work?

- How do you soothe yourself when feeling stressed?

Identify Patterns

Patterns are closely related to themes. They manifest as repeated routines and behaviors that are motivated by thoughts and feelings. For example, if you have a recurring theme of abandonment, you are likely to think that nobody can be trusted or nobody sees and appreciates the real you. These thoughts motivate specific patterns of behaviors that help you navigate relationships with others, which might include being afraid of intimacy, codependent, controlling, and so on. Reflecting, you can trace these behaviors to patterns that are motivated by your beliefs, which are based on recurring themes.

Observe Your Emotional Reactions

Your emotions are clues to determine how various situations impact you. Paying attention to them can help you assess whether your responses are based on reality or history. When your emotions match the actions that are taking place in your environment, they are based on reality. However, when your emotions are blown out of proportion, they are likely triggered by your history.

Once again, you have the opportunity to look for patterns in how you react to certain situations. For example, does the topic of parenting always lead to tearfulness? Do you become angry whenever you sense betrayal or broken trust? Recurring emotional reactions indicate that there is unresolved history that continues to affect how you perceive and respond to present situations.

Write Down Your Thoughts and Feelings

A significant component of shadow work is documenting your thoughts and feelings. Not only does this help you to identify patterns and recurring themes, but it can also help you make sense of your experiences. One of the stumbling blocks that many people face on their road to recovery and healing is figuring out why they do certain things. Their emotional reactions and behaviors remain a mystery due to the lack of introspection and documentation of their experiences.

Furthermore, writing is a form of therapy that assists with decluttering the mind and cultivating self-awareness. It feels as impactful as having a one-on-one session with a therapist. The writing process allows you to release frustration, express sensitive emotions, confront your own demons, and practice telling the truth about your life. The standard form of writing that is supported in shadow work is expressive writing, which entails spontaneously writing down what is on your heart on a piece of paper or notebook without considering spelling, grammar, or any formal structure.

How to Get Started

To ease into the shadow work process, take some time to mentally and physically prepare yourself. Consider whether you have any upcoming events or deadlines that are urgent and must take priority or stressful personal matters that are ongoing and need your full attention to resolve.

Rate your overall well-being out of 10 (with 10 being optimal health). Factor in how much sleep you are getting, the quality of your diet, the stressors you are dealing with, and the amount of time you have to rest and reflect each day. If your rating is below 7 out of 10, dedicate at least a month to adjust your daily routines and improve your wellness.

When you are ready to embark on the shadow work process, start by setting intentions for the journey ahead. Intentions are positive aims that prime your mind to focus on targeted outcomes. Think about what you intend to achieve from going through this process; what personal growth do you hope to experience?

As mentioned in the first chapter, shadow work can be uncomfortable at times, particularly when you are confronted with memories or strong emotions that you were not prepared to encounter. To ensure that you remain dedicated to the process, even when it gets tough, make a few commitments to yourself, such as:

- You will respond to pain with compassion and nonjudgment.

- You will listen to your body and take breaks whenever necessary.

- You will be patient with yourself throughout the shadow work process.

- You will avoid making comparisons with others on a similar healing journey.

- You will be brutally honest about your thoughts and feelings, making no excuses.

- You will prevent shifting blame to others and be responsible for your actions.

- You will seek professional support when the process becomes overwhelming.

- Moreover, there are positive habits that you can incorporate into your daily routine to keep you in the right state of mind to practice shadow work:

- Dedicate at least 10 minutes to practice shadow work.

- Reflect on your moods and performance throughout the day.

- Keep a shadow journal and document your discoveries.

- Practice relaxing stress management techniques during challenging moments.

- Surround yourself with positive influences; avoid people who trigger you.

- Be honest and courageous about how you are feeling in every moment.

- Practice mindfulness in everything you do (e.g., mindful listening, eating, walking).

Shadow work is not a miracle cure that can erase the memory of past experiences. However, the process can reveal personal blind spots that you may have overlooked over the years, which point to the source of your suffering. A good doctor does not prescribe medication before completing a medical diagnosis because they understand that the treatment depends on the unique symptoms that are revealed in the body.

Likewise, shadow work is a psychological and spiritual diagnostic process that focuses on uncovering the root issues behind your unwanted thoughts, emotions, and behaviors. Going into the process, you are encouraged to adopt an open mind so you can go beyond your conscious awareness and dig up unconscious programming that has shaped how you relate with others and the world.

Similar to other forms of therapy, shadow work can trigger repressed thoughts, emotions, and impulses. For many people, this can feel uncomfortable and somewhat counterproductive. Ironically, feeling uncomfortable during the shadow work process is a sign that healing is taking place. To release patterns that are no longer serving you, you must be willing to acknowledge and confront them. If at any point you feel overwhelmed by the experience, feel free to reach out to a psychoanalytic therapist who has training in Jungian psychology and can guide you through the process.

Shadow work is not recommended when you are treating a diagnosed mental health condition or going through a stressful period in your life where your emotions are unstable. The process should not be used as a shortcut to combatting mental illness, breaking bad habits, or learning to manage your time better. These critical issues should be dealt with before you start practicing shadow work so that you have minimal distractions that are preventing you from doing the inner work.

How to Identify Your Shadow

We have mentioned and made examples of one particular way to identify your shadow, which is recognizing emotional triggers. But this particular method isn't the only way. Your shadow can manifest in different ways depending on the present circumstance. Sometimes it can show up as a trigger, other times as an impulse, a thought, or a destructive behavior.

The following list is by no means the full spectrum of how your shadow self can manifest. However, after going through these examples, you will know the clues and patterns to look for when detecting your shadow.

Judging and Criticizing Others

What you cannot accept in yourself is unacceptable in others too. The root of judgment and criticism is personal hang-ups that haven't been acknowledged, explored, and accepted. Seeing these hang-ups displayed in other people's characters and behaviors feels uncomfortable. For example, if you feel pressure to become successful, you might judge people who you perceive as lazy or broke. Seeing their laissez-faire attitude toward money or career progression makes you angry because of how self-critical you are about your own wealth journey.

Playing the Victim

Playing the victim refers to putting yourself in a disempowered position to validate the recurring theme or story about your life. Remember that the shadow self always has an agenda. In this case, the agenda for playing the victim is to elicit sympathy from others. Signs of victimhood include feeling helpless, stranded, and lacking accountability for your actions. These behaviors may have worked in the past to gain favors, attention, or affection from others, which might explain the decision to reenact the behaviors.

Insulting Others and Trolling on the Internet

Taking actions to hurt other people is a manifestation of your shadow. An example of this is posting insulting comments and trolling strangers online. The motivation for this kind of behavior is feeling a sense of pleasure from putting other people down without suffering the consequences. It may also be a way to feel superior or empowered, which makes up for feeling inferior or disempowered in other areas of your life.

Struggles With Setting Strong and Healthy Boundaries

Sometimes the shadow doesn't manifest as aggressive reactions or behaviors but, instead, as passive and pitiful reactions or behaviors. Playing the victim is one of them, and so is struggling to set and enforce strong and healthy boundaries. Letting people walk over you can feel safe for two reasons. First, it enables you to avoid possible conflict and confrontation in expressing your needs. And second, it can be seen as a form of people-pleasing to make others like you or reduce the risk of them abandoning you.

Letting Triggers Get the Best of You

Everybody gets triggered every once in a while. The only time you should be concerned is when a pattern of emotional triggers to specific situations starts to emerge. This is when triggers begin to interfere with your daily functioning or relationships. For example, getting enraged when your teenager forgets to do their chores for the 100th time is understandable. But having the same explosive reaction whenever they so much as look in your direction signals a deeper problem. Something about your parent-child relationship continues to trigger you, and it's deeper than incomplete chores or your child's bad attitude.

Projecting Your Problems Onto Others

Confronting your emotional issues and traumas can cause internalized shame and judgment, which might explain why it takes so long for you to address your problems. Instead of acknowledging your pain, you may decide to make other people responsible for it by projecting your hurt feelings onto them. In the short term, projection brings a sense of relief. However, as time goes on, you can become disillusioned about the root cause of your problems. Projection also creates a cycle of blame and victimhood where you are never responsible for your behaviors.

Abuse of Power

The saying "hurt people hurt people" describes a manifestation of the shadow self. When healing is not an option, the shadow seeks to "make up" for past trauma by inflicting hurt on others. The rationale behind this motivation is, "If I had to endure the pain, why shouldn't they endure it too?" This type of behavior is seen among some people with authority over others, who take their anger out on those under them. They use their power to justify abuse, gain respect through coercion, and aggressively correct the injustices of the past (i.e., targeting people who remind them of their childhood bullies).

Shadow Emotions

Lastly, the shadow can manifest as strong emotions that are perceived as taboo, negative, or inappropriate. They include emotions like anger, fear, envy, disgust, shame, or insecurity. Most times, when these emotions emerge, you will notice the urge to deny, ignore, or suppress them. This is because they make you feel guilty, evil, or not as healed or in control as you might like to think you are.

Shadow emotions are as natural as feeling gratitude and happiness. They are an integral part of your life and necessary for growth. Disowning your shadow emotions creates blindspots that you cannot address, which perpetuates suffering and delays your healing. You don't need to love your shadow emotions to work with them and overcome destructive behaviors. The only thing required is the willingness to withhold judgment so that you can understand the motivation behind them.

There are four simple steps that you can practice to identify and embrace your shadow emotions:

Step 1: Label What You Are Feeling

The fear of emotions stems from ignorance about your emotional experiences. When you understand your emotions and have the vocabulary to name and describe your feelings, you gain control over your emotional experience. Moreover, you can separate yourself from your emotional experiences to show that you are not what you feel. Practice looking up synonyms and dictionary definitions of emotions to learn the nuances of your emotional experiences. Instead of using a word that you are familiar with like anger, find another word that gets close to the kind of anger you are feeling, such as irritation or resentment.

Step 2: Observe Your Triggered Thoughts

Your shadow emotions are fueled by thoughts that justify their existence. These are negative thoughts that distort your perception of what's taking place in reality. The thoughts can be directed at you, other people, or the current situation. Furthermore, they can come to your mind as bold statements or audible voices of your inner critic or people from your past who were judgmental. For example, after a binge on sugar foods, you might feel ashamed of yourself (shadow emotion) and hear the voice of your mother saying, "You are so fat!" Remain calm and take deep breaths to de-escalate the trigger and prevent further destructive choices.

Step 3: Let Go of Judgment

This next step is crucial for managing shadow emotions. Instead of reacting to your thoughts and feelings (which is the natural human instinct), practice riding the wave. Sit still and do nothing as you allow the unpleasant experience to continue its course until it comes to an end. If you struggle to manage your urges, delay your reaction for five minutes, then another five minutes, until the motivation to act on your urges has gone.

Another strategy that can help you let go of judgment is taking the opposite action. If your default is to judge, practice radical acceptance of how you feel. Recite the famous Hawaiian Ho'oponopono mantra that says, "I'm sorry, please forgive me, thank you, I love you" (Williamson, 2019).

Step 4: Embrace Your Shadow Emotions

When judgment is placed aside, acceptance is invited. At this stage, you are not concerned about how terrible the emotions are, who might judge you for displaying the emotions, and any other cognitive or social pressure that was standing in the way of fully embracing your shadow emotions. You can accept that shadow emotions are genuine representations of how you might feel in the moment, even though they don't define who you are. Similar to welcoming guests into your home, you know that they will leave at some point, and you will return to normal operations.

Embracing your shadow emotions is not about loving them or agreeing with your negative reactions. It is about allowing yourself to go through pleasant and unpleasant experiences without making yourself feel bad. With this level of openness toward your emotional experiences, you can see them as teachable moments rather than shameful displays of weakness. You are capable of bouncing back from shadow emotions, but only when you see the potential to learn and grow from them.

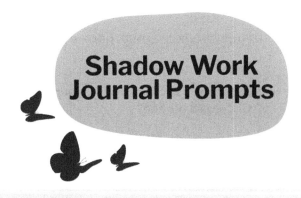

Shadow Work Journal Prompts

1. What is the significance of going through the shadow work process for you?

2. What are you most and least looking forward to on the shadow work journey?

3. If you were to describe the current themes of your life, what would they be?

4. What unhealthy coping mechanisms do you hope to explore and challenge?

5. Describe at least three recurring situations that consistently provoke your emotional triggers.

6. Describe at least three people who consistently provoke your emotional triggers.

7. What shadow emotions arise before and during your emotional triggers?

8. How would you describe your relationship with your shadow emotions?

9. Reflect on a humiliating situation as a child. What happened? Who was there? What about the situation caused you to feel humiliated?

10. Reflect on a humiliating situation as an adult. What happened? Who was there? What about the situation caused you to feel humiliated?

11. Would you describe yourself as someone who is self-critical? If so, in what ways do you criticize yourself?

12. Do you remember being criticized as a child? If so, who were the people who criticized you, and what kind of things would they say?

13. If you were to describe your inner critical voice, what would it sound like?

14. How has the emotion of shame manifested in your life?

15. When was the first time you remember feeling like you were not good enough?

16. Which aspects of your identity do you associate with weakness?

17. Which aspects of your identity do you associate with strength?

18. What compliment have you received from someone that you struggle to believe?

19. What privilege do you have that you don't believe you deserve?

20. Have you ever entertained the idea of living a different reality?

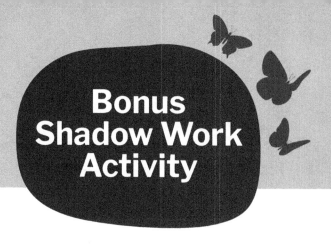

Bonus Shadow Work Activity

Intuitive Drawing

Grab a sheet of paper and craft supplies, and find a quiet place where you can draw. The goal of intuitive drawing is to connect with your unconscious self and spontaneously illustrate your shadow.

To get your creative juices flowing, here are a few helpful tips:

• Draw a picture of yourself using your less dominant hand (i.e., left hand if your right hand is dominant).

• Use colors as a symbolic representation of your emotions.

• Draw with your eyes closed to prevent judgment of your artwork

• Remember to reflect on and analyze your drawing when you have completed it. With a nonjudgmental eye, look at what you have drawn and connect to the significance behind the art. Ask yourself open-ended questions like:

• What inspired you to create this artwork?

• Reflect on your use of colors, shapes, and text.

• What thoughts or emotions came up while completing this exercise?

• Were there any physical or mental challenges you experienced?

• What is the takeaway message from your drawing? What does your shadow want you to know?

Preparation is critical to getting the most out of your shadow work journey. Now that you are familiar with the process and basic practices, we can proceed to the next chapter and discuss ways to manage emotional disturbances that might come.

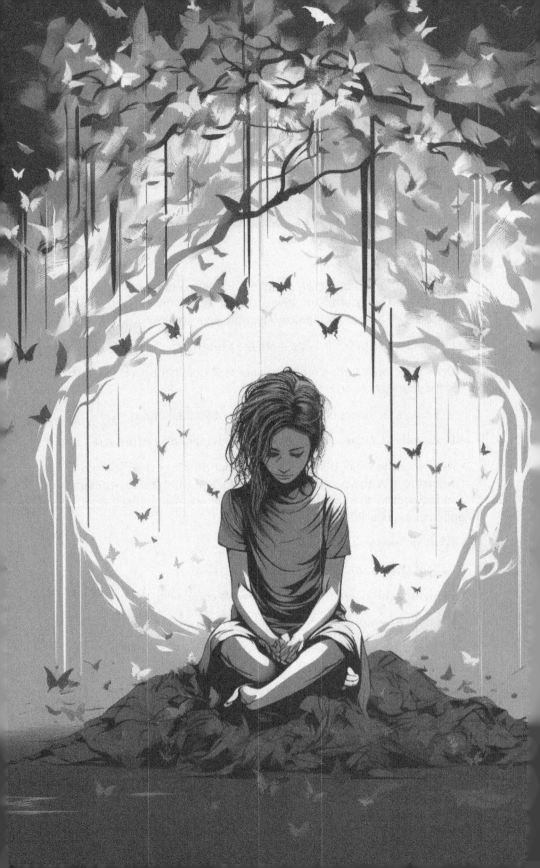

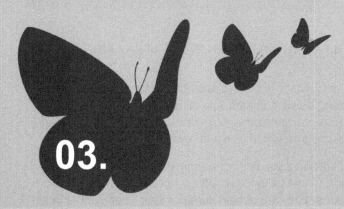

03.

Navigating Inevitable Emotional Turbulence

Your Shadow is all of the things, "positive" and "negative," that you've denied about yourself and hidden beneath the surface of the mask you forgot that you're wearing. –Oli Anderson

Unpleasant Emotions During Shadow Work

Your psyche is programmed to seek pleasure and avoid pain. This instinctual mechanism is partly responsible for your survival. The risk of exposing yourself to pain is that it can potentially damage your mind and body to the point of no return, hence why you are motivated to stay in your comfort zone and avoid risky or life-threatening situations.

Shadow work and other forms of therapy that promote psychological healing access your subconscious mind and bring up painful memories and traumas that you have neglected. Since your brain perceives what you are thinking and feeling as experiences that are taking place right now, recalling painful memories and traumas triggers the body's fight-flight-freeze response and creates emotional distress, as though you were reliving the past.

Even though your life is not endangered when you are reflecting on the past, it certainly feels so. Recalling painful experiences can cause physical symptoms like migraines, stomach pain, shortness of breath, and muscle tension, similar to someone who is in a life-threatening situation.

Naturally, your human instinct will be to stop the shadow work process and go back to shutting down, numbing, and distracting yourself with less stressful activities. However, going this route blocks you from confronting, accepting, and releasing unresolved pain and trauma.

The unpleasant emotions that you feel during shadow work are a necessary component of healing. Some of these emotions have been stored in your body for many decades. They are behind some of your negative thinking patterns, irrational fears, and psychological blockages that have become normalized. The reason why they hadn't bothered you in the past is that they were hidden in your subconscious mind. To process and release them, you must be able to sit with the heaviness and darkness that may surface.

Society conditions us to accept pleasurable emotions and reject unpleasant ones. This dates back to moral and religious views of good and evil, whereby good people are seen not to have any dark traits or desires. Recently, the New Age positivity movement has also promoted an idealistic state of ongoing happiness that can be achieved by reprogramming the mind. While it is possible to consciously choose positive thoughts and emotions, it doesn't eradicate the unconscious self, which cannot easily be controlled.

In other words, human beings have a dualistic nature that encompasses both light and darkness. We cannot accept the light without accepting the darkness too. Embracing our dualistic nature makes accepting unpleasant emotions feel less offensive because we know that pain comes with pleasure. Moreover, being open to experiencing discomfort creates opportunities for personal enrichment and growth. We get to understand our multifaceted human nature and discover our innate abilities to transform pain into wisdom.

Blogger Callum Asylab tells the story of how shadow work helped to improve his mental health. For many years, he battled with anxiety and depression but didn't know what was causing it. Initially, he thought that the tireless working hours as a nurse were the main culprit behind his mental illness. However, the symptoms didn't go away after switching up his routine, changing his diet, and adopting practices like reciting positive affirmations. One day, he stumbled on video lessons of Carl Jung explaining the shadow. He found the content interesting, so he did more in-depth research and eventually began the shadow work process.

Confronting the truth about who he was and how his life had played out was an emotional roller-coaster. He remembers journaling with tears dripping on the page and smudging the ink. The heaviness that was buried deep inside his subconscious mind came out in waves of anger. The more open he was to the experience, the more pain could resurface and flow out. Throughout the process, Callum would ask himself "why" to dig up layers and layers of trauma and get closer to wholeness. Every time he would challenge himself by asking "why," he felt strong emotions riling up. Nevertheless, he courageously continued to get to the root of the emotional wounds. By embracing his unpleasant emotions, Callum was able to discover more of himself and address a mental illness that had festered for many years.

When I started asking myself 'why' and started to feel my inner emotions rile up, I dug deeper into that hurt, pain, and anxiety I was told to shut off... I felt liberated and realized: if this could help me, then maybe it could help others. (Asylab, 2023)

How to Handle Resistance

Resistance is an overwhelming feeling that arises whenever there are split internal motivations. For instance, a part of you may desire to dig deeper and explore an unconscious behavior, but there is another part of you that hesitates to do so.

Feeling resistance is a sign of positive growth. It means that there is an aspect of you, let's call it the "wise self," that has emerged and desires to break free from the cognitive and psychological patterns that you have maintained for many years. The wise self is curious and confident and knows that there is so much more that you haven't discovered about yourself. It seeks to steer you toward the direction of change but gets prevented by your ego self.

Your ego self is the aspect of you that justifies your existence. It is the persona that you think and feel that you are. The ego self is who you refer to as "I," the fixed personality that you rely on to make decisions, interpret the world, and judge human behavior. The ego is self-centered, meaning that it is primarily concerned about its survival. It is afraid of change or embracing the unknown because of how it might be impacted.

The clash between the wise self and the ego self creates internal resistance. Overcoming the resistance empowers your wise self, but succumbing to the resistance empowers your ego self. To overcome resistance and empower your wise self, you must acknowledge whether you are experiencing conscious or unconscious resistance and identify the underlying motivations.

Conscious Resistance

Conscious resistance is a feeling of being opposed to something that you are aware of. It often appears whenever you are about to step outside of your comfort zone, pursue goals, or make decisions you have identified as good for you. For example, the day before a job interview, you might feel opposed to attending the meeting. The thought of sitting down with the recruiter and being asked questions could make you feel sick to your stomach. If you make the mistake of attaching to this feeling rather than simply observing it, you might convince yourself to postpone the interview and potentially miss the opportunity.

The motivation behind conscious resistance is the deep-rooted need to defend yourself against potential threats, manipulation, or suspicious behaviors. This defensive response can be traced back to your childhood when you felt the need to put up a defense against controlling parents, school bullies, judgmental people, or anyone whom you felt didn't have your best interests at heart. Back then, resisting their support, guidance, or behaviors made you feel safe and in control. However, as an adult, this internalized and unregulated defensive response manifests as rebellion for the sake of being rebellious and carrying out unconscious acts of self-sabotage.

Healing conscious resistance can be done in two ways, as described next.

Acknowledge the Resistance

Whenever you feel the urge to pull back, doubt, or judge something that you have identified as being good for you, take a moment to pause. Tune in to your body and embrace what you are feeling. You will notice sensations of stress or anxiety or feeling deeply overwhelmed. This is the emergence of conscious resistance. Remind yourself that you are not placing yourself in danger by pursuing the opportunity. Speak to that little girl or boy who may still feel suspicious of people or new experiences and reassure them that there is nothing for them to worry about.

Redefine Your Beliefs

Every time conscious resistance emerges, see this as an opportunity to clarify your beliefs about safety, trust, and change. In most cases, these are the underlying motivations for your defensive responses. Reflect on your current beliefs and assumptions about safety, trust, and change. Consider how they might be blocking you from embracing new experiences and self-actualizing. Be curious about what your life would look like if you redefined these beliefs and assumptions to allow for greater freedom and exploration.

For example, you might feel conscious resistance every time you get to know a person romantically and get to the stage of developing intimacy. You may feel resistant because of underlying trust issues and having a few run-ins with manipulative people in the past. Therefore, it feels safer to simply reject them or maintain emotional distance to avoid being hurt or disappointed.

Once you have acknowledged the resistance, you can redefine your beliefs about trust. Instead of thinking, "Nobody can be trusted," you might entertain the idea that "Trust is earned." This alternative belief creates enough room to get to know acquaintances without being blocked by the fear of being taken for granted. Thus, you can overcome conscious resistance and develop relationships where trust can be built through affirming behaviors.

Unconscious Resistance

Unconscious resistance is a form of opposition that feels out of your control. Imagine that you have decided to start saving toward purchasing a property and then end up with a massive financial crisis to attend to. You may start to feel like whenever you make an effort to change your life for the better, something always gets in the way.

This form of resistance often appears as a self-fulfilling prophecy. It is the product of having split motivations and going back and forth between the wise self and ego self. Even though it may seem as though you are manifesting your worst nightmare, the truth is that you are manifesting something that you unconsciously support or believe.

A good example of this is having a goal to lose weight. The formula for weight loss is straightforward: burn more calories than you consume. This means eating healthier foods and staying active each week. However, many times, unconscious resistance gets in the way and creates all kinds of obstacles that delay or sabotage the process, such as lack of motivation, increased work demands, unexplained sickness, or procrastination.

Whenever you suspect that there may be external forces sabotaging you, examine whether you are manifesting unconscious resistance. It may be uncomfortable to think that you are your own worst enemy, the person standing in front of your success; however, confronting this truth can bring enlightenment and end the unconscious sabotage.

Visualize the presence of two internal forces—the wise self and ego self—fighting for the power seat in your mind. The wise self wants you to outgrow unproductive patterns and habits and mature into a better version of yourself. The ego self is threatened by change and prefers to stick to what has always worked in the past. The closer you come to facing your fears, the more inner conflict you will feel. This is part of the journey to personal growth. Whenever you feel frightened by what you desire, ask yourself: *What are the benefits of pursuing this desire? What kinds of beliefs support this experience?*

Tips for Embracing Vulnerability

Vulnerability is the courage to be sensitive and emotionally expressive. It requires you to let down your psychological defenses and be seen by others. Vulnerability toward yourself entails being honest about your needs, emotions, mistakes, and the impact of previous life experiences.

There are emotional risks that come with embracing vulnerability, which explains why many people choose not to. For instance, when you express emotional needs to a loved one, you run the risk of being misunderstood. Or when you decide to admit your mistakes, you run the risk of feeling like a failure. There are always two outcomes waiting on the other side of vulnerability: acceptance or rejection. Embracing the fear of rejection builds courage and enables you to take emotional risks.

Vulnerability is the gateway to expressing your authentic self. It gives you the confidence to be honest with yourself about your life experiences and remain resilient during challenging moments. Vulnerability can enhance the quality of your relationships and promote healthier communication. Instead of being defensive when you cannot agree with others or when you feel attacked by them, you can acknowledge and describe the frustration and articulate what you need to feel safe and nurtured.

Vulnerability can also improve your relationship with yourself, particularly when it comes to embracing your shadow and showing compassion for your flaws. Here are three examples of how being vulnerable can assist in your shadow work:

- When you feel the pressure to hide or adjust aspects of yourself to gain acceptance from a group, vulnerability helps you present the authentic version of yourself and share your thoughts and opinions, accepting the possibility of being disliked.

• When you are entering a new romantic relationship, vulnerability helps you be honest about your needs and expectations as well as transparent about your boundaries.

• When you have experienced a setback, vulnerability helps you process the disappointment of not achieving what you wanted and talk about your mistakes and the lessons you will take away from the experience.

Traditional societies do not promote vulnerability because it is perceived as a sign of weakness. Little boys and girls who embrace their sensitive sides are often bullied, which causes them to hide their vulnerability deep inside the unconscious mind. The vulnerability appears as a manifestation of their shadow selves, something that is bad and embarrassing rather than something to be celebrated. As a result, their reactions to feeling vulnerable are to lash out in anger, blame others, go into isolation, or numb themselves with substances. This can be traced back to toxic social conditioning (e.g., "Real men don't cry") and being denied their right to feel emotions.

Here are some tips that you can follow to practice embracing vulnerability instead of running away from it:

• **Practice kindness toward yourself.** Notice how you speak to yourself or respond to your pain. Decide on a loving role that you can play (e.g., mentor, parent, friend) to help you cultivate self-love. Remind yourself that you deserve kindness and understanding as much as the next person.

• **Let go of seeking to prove your worth.** Learn to validate yourself by your growth, goals, and mindset. Accept the fact that not everybody will appreciate who you are or provide the support you are looking for. Have the courage to continue expressing your authentic self, even when others disapprove.

• **Don't expect miracles from yourself.** Part of practicing self-love is learning to be patient with your growth. Set realistic expectations that help you improve without putting you under pressure. Make time for self-care in between work to balance your needs and give your body a chance to reset and recharge.

• **Avoid perfectionism.** Let go of the pressure to be perfect and take an honest appraisal of your strengths and weaknesses. Be humble enough to admit that you don't know everything and, therefore, need guidance to become a better version of yourself.

- **Be honest with your needs.** Remind yourself that having needs does not make you a needy person. Sharing your needs gives other people the opportunity to show love and support. Those who genuinely love you desire to take care of you; however, they need instructions to respond to your needs.

- **Share your feelings.** Your emotions are valid and help those around you understand how you perceive the world. Sharing your feelings gives other people insight into who you are and what you need. This courageous act can also strengthen your relationships by creating an emotional connection.

- **Practice living in the moment.** Shift your focus to the present moment and embrace the thoughts and emotions that arise. Being present requires vulnerability because you are encouraged to accept reality (as peaceful or chaotic as it may be) instead of entertaining fantasies.

What to Do When Unpleasant Emotions Surface

Imagine that your body is a large steel pot placed on a hot stove, and the unpleasant emotion is boiling water. As the temperature of the water gets hotter, does the pot melt under pressure? No. It remains solid and unchangeable. The resistance you feel when unpleasant emotions surface can be mild and tolerable or intense and overwhelming. However, your body is strong enough to handle the pressure. With that said, you need to be equipped with the proper coping mechanisms to manage your emotions effectively so you can uncover the wounds behind them instead of being tempted to push them down.

The following set of steps will help you work through difficult emotions and identify and manage emotional triggers. You will also find tips that introduce you to healthy coping mechanisms to manage difficult emotions and triggers.

Four Steps to Work Through Difficult Emotions

This four-step process of working through difficult emotions is based on a technique introduced by clinical psychologist Dr. Beth Kurland. In her practice, she noticed that many of her clients avoided or felt helpless whenever difficult emotions would arise. To help them cope with these intense emotions, she suggested an exercise called "seeking shade," where one invites a more expansive emotion to coexist and sit alongside the difficult emotion one struggles to accept (Kurland, 2022). For example, if you are feeling lonely, you might invite a feeling of acceptance. If you are angry, you might invite understanding. Seeking shade makes it easier to cope with your difficult emotions without resisting or trying to change your circumstances.

Follow these four steps to learn how to seek shade:

Step 1: Identify the Difficult Emotion

Name the problematic emotion you are feeling. Acknowledge its presence and how nuanced it is. For example, the primary emotion you might feel is anger, but it manifests as being dismissive. In a single sentence, describe how you are feeling. You might say, "I feel myself being dismissive because I am angry and don't feel like talking right now."

Step 2: Ask Yourself: What Would Help Me Feel Ease During This Emotion?

Consider how you can improve the moment by inviting an expansive emotion. This is the part where you seek shade. It can help to imagine a loved one noticing how you are feeling and asking how they can balance or bring ease to what you are feeling. Note that the expansive emotion is not the opposite of what you are currently experiencing but, instead, more uplifting. For example, compassion uplifts self-criticism, and patience uplifts anxiety. What would uplift your difficult emotion?

Step 3: Think of a Time When the Expansive Emotion Improved Your Situation

Go into your mental files and recall a time in the past when the expansive emotions you are inviting improved the outcome of a situation. For instance, if you are inviting understanding to coexist with frustration, you might recall a time when putting yourself in another person's shoes brought more clarity to the situation. You may want to journal your response for this step to unpack what happened and explain the positive impact your expansive emotion made on the situation.

Step 4: Visualize and Invite the Expansive Emotion

Visualization is a technique that involves creating mental imagery to invoke a state of being or envision a desired outcome. Using this technique, create a mental image of the expansive emotion and envision it entering your body through deep breathing (i.e., breathe in the expansive emotion and breathe out the difficult emotion) or surrounding your body like a warm and loving force field of light. Another idea is to imagine the expansive emotion in the sky, and your difficult emotions are passing clouds. The goal here is to notice the "bigness" of your expansive emotion and how it can support you in this current state.

Eight Steps to Identify and Manage Emotional Triggers

Emotional triggers are slightly different from difficult emotions in that they are rapid impulses that occur in a matter of seconds but promote explosive reactions and destructive habits. There are two ways to cope with emotional triggers: prevent them from occurring by identifying them early or manage them gracefully when they are fully active. Here are four steps that will help you identify emotional triggers and four steps to help you manage them.

Follow these steps to identify your emotional triggers:

Step 1: Tune Into Your Mind and Body

Your mind and body will give you warning signals to alert you of incoming triggers. Pay attention to physiological and psychological changes that are out of the ordinary. Physical symptoms might include rapid heart rate, difficulty breathing, sweating, gut issues, or trouble concentrating. Psychological symptoms might include irritability, anxiety, taking offense, or having an out-of-body experience. If you are not attuned to your body sensations, practice tracking your moods and physical sensations daily. This will help you gauge your normal responses, making it easier to pick up on changes.

Step 2: Stop Everything You Are Doing and Take a Step Back

Once you have identified changes to your physiology or psychology, resist the temptation to dig deeper. Take a step back and physically or emotionally distance yourself from the situation. This break in thinking and taking action is necessary to regulate your nervous system, which is responsible for your fight-flight-freeze responses. It can also turn off the primitive part of your brain that is known to be impulsive and activate your prefrontal cortex, which is in charge of logic and reasoning.

Step 3: Trace the Roots of Your Discomfort

At this stage, you are feeling inner discomfort that hasn't yet formed into a trigger. To reverse the process, identify what happened that made you feel this way. Could it have been words spoken by a colleague? An offensive TV commercial? Anxiety about an upcoming deadline? Or receiving bad news over the phone? Go a step further and trace back the discomfort to an experience where a similar situation took place. For example, if you felt uncomfortable being disciplined by your manager, you may have a history of not getting along with your employers.

Step 4: Get Curious

If the connection between your discomfort and the situation at hand is not clear, spend time reflecting on your experience to uncover why your body reacted in that manner. Exercises like meditation and journaling can be useful when seeking to explore your subconscious mind. Remember that your mind and body respond to ingrained patterns. Get curious about discovering the pattern that led you to feel stressed in that particular situation.

Sometimes, you may not be able to catch your triggers before they kick off. Don't worry; the following steps will show you how to manage them gracefully without leading to explosive reactions.

Step 1: Embrace Your Emotions With Openness

Emotions are not bad or good, they are signals or messages that help you understand how you are feeling in the moment. Acknowledge the strong emotions that have emerged and where they are situated in your body. Accept them for what they are without judging the appropriateness. If you feel angry, sit with the emotion without trying to change it. Practice the "seeking shade" exercise to cope with your emotions.

Step 2: Create Room to Breathe

Give yourself the space to process what you are feeling by either standing up and walking away from the triggering situation or turning inward and practicing deep breathing and grounding techniques. The aim is to gradually calm your nervous system and return to a normal state of mind. Creating room to breathe is also about nurturing yourself through the difficult moment. Be honest about what you need that could improve the moment. For example, do you need to postpone a contentious meeting at work? Do you need to isolate yourself in your bedroom for 15 minutes?

Step 3: Maintain an Open Mind

If your emotional trigger was caused by a situation involving other people, don't be quick to make assumptions about what might have happened. How you perceive the situation is only one side of the story. What additional information might you be overlooking? It is easy to misinterpret another person's behaviors when you don't understand their intention. Perhaps asking questions can help you get closer to the truth about what happened. You may find that you were not the only person triggered by the situation.

Step 4: Have an Honest Conversation

When you are emotionally triggered and feeling vulnerable, the last thing you want to do is open yourself up again and communicate your feelings. However, taking this courageous step can help you maintain strong relationships that do not need repair after every disagreement or misunderstanding. Having open and honest conversations can also set a precedence for how to resolve conflict in the future. This can create an emotionally safe space to share your experiences without feeling afraid of what the other person might say.

Lead with "I" statements to show ownership of your thoughts and feelings and avoid making accusations. After expressing what you felt and the thoughts that crossed your mind, give the other person an opportunity to respond and set the record straight. If you need an apology, ask for one. If a boundary is required, enforce one. Use the conversation as an outlet to heal and bounce back stronger from the situation.

The steps mentioned above may not be sufficient to help you cope with difficult emotions or emotional triggers, particularly if there is trauma involved. Signs that you need to seek professional help include not being able to complete tasks, regulate your moods, maintain healthy relationships without conflict, or carry out everyday functions due to emotional instability.

Coping Mechanisms to Manage Difficult Emotions in the Moment

In addition to seeking support from a mental health professional, here are effective ways to manage difficult emotions in the moment:

- **Be mindful of your thoughts.** Keep a close watch on your thoughts, particularly negative ideas or beliefs that intensify your emotions. Many times, these thoughts seem justifiable or consoling, but they lead you down a path of suffering. Specifically, look out for assumptions or generalizations that are based on opinions or emotions instead of indisputable facts.

- **Put a name to the emotion.** As mentioned earlier, naming what you are feeling gives you more control over the emotion and helps you create distance between you and what you are experiencing. Not only are you able to get a wider perspective of your emotion, but you also have options about how to respond to it.

72

- **Get active and exercise.** Physical exercise is a great stress reliever and mood enhancer. When you are feeling overwhelmed, engaging in light or moderate exercises can serve as a positive distraction and release endorphins, which make you feel good.

- **Have a sense of humor about it.** Laughing at yourself can reduce emotional pain and shift how you think about the troubling situation. Having a sense of humor doesn't discredit what you are feeling or going through; it simply reminds you to embrace the present moment and feel gratitude for the small things in life.

- **Prioritize self-care.** When you are feeling emotional discomfort, that is your cue to check in with yourself and address underlying needs. Think of small and meaningful ways to make yourself feel better through acts of self-care. What is your strong emotion calling for? Self-care does not need to be over-the-top because your needs are basic and uncomplicated. Getting an extra hour of sleep can be exactly what you need to feel rejuvenated in the morning.

- **Make to-do lists.** Poor time management and organizational skills can make you feel like you are not in control of your life. Take your power back by getting into the habit of writing down and prioritizing your tasks. Start with the most important tasks that bring the most value, then slowly get through the others. If you are overwhelmed by the number of tasks, consider which ones you can delegate, postpone, or cancel out.

- **Set healthy boundaries.** Healthy boundaries are limits that protect you from overcommitting yourself or dishonoring your needs and values. In most cases, being on the receiving end of bad behavior gives you the perfect opportunity to set a boundary. When doing so, start by describing the situation, focusing on the behavior you cannot accept. Thereafter, express the emotional impact of such behavior and specify what you need to change moving forward. Be direct about the consequences that might follow if the same mistakes are repeated in the future.

Coping Mechanisms to Face Emotional Triggers

The emotional trigger has kicked off. You can feel a whirlpool of emotions gaining more strength inside of you. The urge to fight or take flight is becoming intense by the minute. You panic and wonder if it's too late to turn the situation around. The good news is that it isn't too late to regain control of your emotional triggers once they have fully formed and taken over your body.

An effective practice that you can adopt is mind therapy borrowed from the Eastern tradition, commonly known as mindfulness.

Mindfulness refers to the practice of being present in the moment. The purpose of this is to end the suffering caused by overthinking, catastrophizing, and creating stories about what is happening at the moment. The truth is that reality is never as painful as the mind paints it out to be. However, you can only realize this by shifting your focus to the present moment. Emotional triggers are fueled by impulses and thoughts. Once you let go of the thoughts, you will find it easier to manage the impulses that are rushing through your body at this moment.

Another way to practice mindfulness is to observe the trigger without feeling compelled to act on it. Imagine that you are standing outside of your body and watching yourself have an emotional experience. Notice how the trigger starts and progresses and the different physiological changes that occur. Continue to watch as the trigger loses momentum and your body gradually returns to a normal state.

What makes mindfulness effective in managing emotional triggers is that the practice promotes emotional awareness. You get to practice accepting and sitting with a range of emotions without feeling intimidated or overwhelmed by them. Furthermore, when resistance emerges (which it often does), you can also observe and accept the resistance without forming a story or identifying with it.

At the end of the day, your thoughts, emotions, and resistance are merely energy that is generated inside of you, which can be guided and channeled in any direction. Mindfulness seeks to create a space where the energy can flow without being contained or suppressed. Eventually, the energy will naturally lose power and return to nothingness or flow out of your body.

Since emotional triggers create strong impulses, it is essential to avoid turning to unhealthy coping mechanisms that promote addictive habits and behaviors. Examples of unhealthy coping mechanisms include overeating, binge drinking, self-medicating, sleeping excessively, venting your problems to others, or avoiding your problems altogether. All the behaviors mentioned feel good at the moment; however, in the long run, they can create new problems that complicate your life.

Avoidance of emotional pain does not make the pain go away. It simply delays your healing process. Healthy coping mechanisms don't numb your pain because numbing leads to avoidance. Instead, they are designed to reduce the symptoms of pain and clear your head space so you can confront your problems.

Dive into Transformation with Your Review: Embrace the Shadows, Embrace Yourself

"Money can't buy happiness, but discovering your hidden depths can." - Anonymous

People who explore the depths of their being often find richer lives and deeper connections with others. So, let's take a plunge into the unknown together.

Here's a question for you: Would you help someone on their journey of self-discovery, even if no one knew it was you?

Who is this person, you wonder? They are much like you, or perhaps how you once were—seeking understanding, craving growth, and yearning for change, but uncertain where to start.

Our quest is to share the wisdom of *Transformative Shadow Work* with all who seek it. Everything we do is guided by this mission. And the only way to fulfill it is by reaching... well... everyone.

That's where you step in. As much as we may deny it, many of us do judge a book by its cover (and its reviews). So here's my humble request on behalf of a fellow seeker you've never crossed paths with.

Please lend your voice by leaving a review for this book.

To experience the joy of making a difference and truly aiding another seeker, it's as simple as this, taking less than a minute:

Scan the QR code to leave your review:

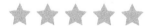

If the notion of helping an anonymous seeker resonates with you, then you're exactly the kind of person I admire. Welcome to the club. You're one of us.

I'm even more thrilled to guide you through your journey to self-discovery and acceptance. You'll find the insights within the pages ahead to be invaluable.

With heartfelt gratitude, let's continue our shared voyage.

Your devoted guide, Lulu Nicholson.

Shadow Work Journal Prompts

1. Name and describe an emotion that makes you feel uneasy.

2. Think back to your childhood. How did you manage stress?

3. Was there an emotion you were discouraged from feeling as a child?

4. What negative emotion have you normalized or treated as a part of your day-to-day experience?

5. What memories from your childhood make you feel ashamed?

6. What memories from your childhood make you feel powerless?

7. In what ways do you self-sabotage yourself? Think of at least three scenarios related to your career, health, and relationships.

8. How important are you to yourself? Have you always been encouraged to prioritize your well-being?

9. Have you ever made decisions to make other people happy? Why?

10. How open are you to trying new experiences?

11. How do you respond to unexpected changes?

12. What do you fear the most about outgrowing your current way of life?

13. You are aware of the benefits of healing. Now explore the disadvantages. What will you lose as a result of healing? How will that affect your life?

14. Reflect on the younger versions of yourself. Which period of your life are you least proud of? Why?

15. Are you still carrying guilt about something that happened years ago? If so, what has made it difficult to let go of the guilt?

16. What do you need to forgive yourself for? In what ways have you betrayed yourself?

**17. In what ways are you showing up for others that
you need to start practicing toward yourself?**

**18. What positive emotions do you frequently downplay
out of fear of losing control or being judged?**

19. Do you feel worthy of genuine, unconditional love? Why?

20. How can you be more gentle and compassionate with yourself throughout the shadow work process? Mention a few suggestions.

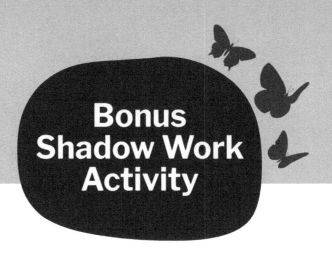

Bonus Shadow Work Activity

Shadow Work Meditation

You may be familiar with the practice of meditation, another effective mind therapy borrowed from Eastern tradition. If mindfulness is about being present in the moment, meditation encourages you to connect with the deepest parts of yourself. Shadow work meditation seeks to heal and embrace your shadow by exploring and holding space for your unpleasant thoughts, memories, and emotions.

Of course, this process doesn't happen over one session but across several meditation sessions. Shadow work meditation can help you regulate your emotions, come to terms with negative past experiences, and reach a place of forgiveness and acceptance. By allowing your unresolved emotional issues to come to the surface and being willing to greet them with acceptance, they no longer become something that you fear or feel ashamed about.

The internet is full of powerful shadow work guided meditations that you can browse through. Below is a simple script that you can practice to get familiar with the process. Remember that standard meditation rules apply. For best results, find a quiet room where you can spend uninterrupted time by yourself. Sit in a comfortable position and spend a few minutes regulating and slowing down your breathing before you start. If you start feeling overwhelmed during the meditation, gently shift your attention to your breathing and return to the script when you have stabilized your emotions.

Meditation Script

Bring to your mind a recent or ongoing situation that is causing moderate stress. This could be a situation related to your health, work, family, and so on. Replay the situation in your mind from beginning to end.

Remind yourself of how it started, progressed, and has developed or been resolved. Consider the emotional impact of the situation, how it has made you feel, or what past traumas it has triggered.

Now that the experience is alive in your mind, connect with your body. Notice how your body responds to the recollection of the story. Where along your body do you feel discomfort? What does the discomfort feel like? Continue to be present with the sensations flowing through your body.

With the situation still playing in your mind, repeat the following statement to yourself at least three times:

- **"This is a moment of struggling."** Validate your emotional discomfort by embracing the feeling. Acknowledge how difficult it may feel to sit with your emotions. Be mindful of the fact that you are in pain, but remind yourself that the pain is temporary and will surely pass.

- **"Struggle is a part of life."** Realize that you are not alone in experiencing this kind of pain. Many people across the world are dealing with similar struggles. Find comfort in the fact that you share this experience with billions of people who have been through and overcome this moment of suffering.

- **"May I accept myself as I am."** Place your hand on your chest and repeat these compassionate words to yourself. Feel the safety and warmth of your hand and take a moment to appreciate the support that you offer yourself.

Emotional turbulence is inevitable during the shadow work process, but the upside is that feeling emotional pain and finding healthy ways to cope and manage the experience encourages you to become a reliable source of support for yourself.

We have now completed the first part of the book where we took a deep dive into the concept and fundamentals of shadow work. You have been equipped with the necessary tools and skills to proceed to the second part of the book, which takes you through the journey of shadow work.

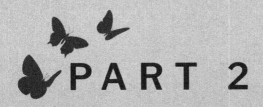

PART 2

UNDERSTANDING SHADOW WORK

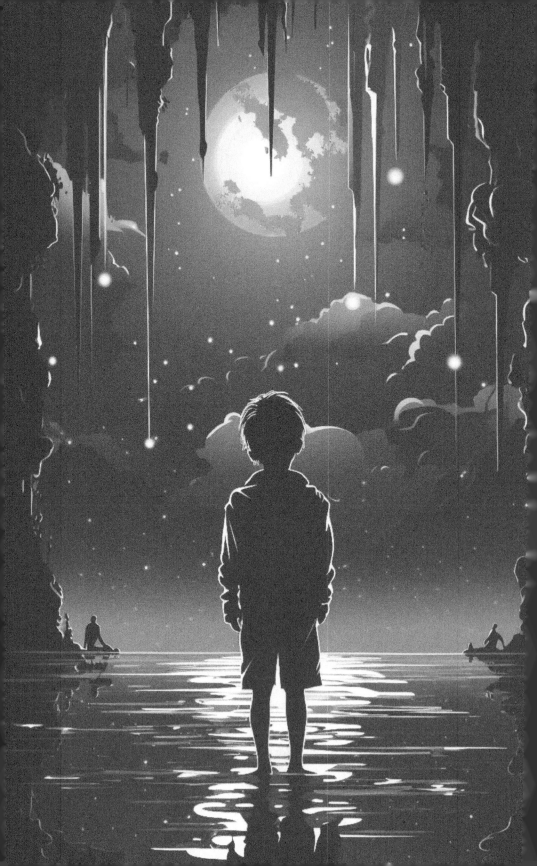

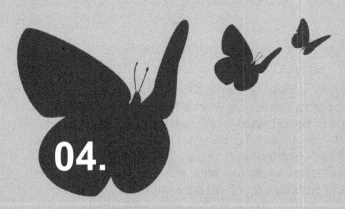

04.

Starting Your Trauma Recovery Journey

I used to live my life at night in the shadow of my dark past, I lived in shadows for so long until the dark became my world, but then you came and flipped on a light, at first I was blinded, it was so bright, but over time my eyes adjusted and I could see and now what's in focus is our future, bright, brighter than it's ever been. –Danny Maximus

Recognizing the Impact of Past Trauma

Trauma is the psychological response to an event or series of events that have caused a significant amount of stress. Experiences like losing a loved one, getting in a car accident, being terminally ill, or succumbing to violence and abuse can contribute to the development of trauma. How experiences are perceived and processed can also lead to trauma. For example, a child who feels emotionally neglected by her parents or an adult whose unemployment status makes him feel inadequate can develop trauma wounds.

With that being said, not everyone who has gone through hardships and difficult moments in life will develop trauma. Since trauma is a psychological response, it is triggered by certain thoughts, beliefs, and emotions. The particular event or series of events must be perceived as life-threatening and beyond the individual's control for them to feel stressed, insecure, anxious, and hopeless.

Trauma can manifest during or immediately after a threatening situation, or the symptoms can appear years later. The initial reaction to trauma is shock due to the difficulty of processing the experience. As the shock wears off—which can take many months or years—survivors may feel confused, in denial, agitated, or numb. They may also begin to regain consciousness of what they have been through, which can trigger overwhelming emotions that have been suppressed during this time. These emotions can resurface at once or in waves and cause a mental health disorder called post-traumatic stress disorder (PTSD).

The symptoms of trauma take longer to process and release compared to the time it takes to acknowledge and come to terms with the traumatic incident. Many survivors will report accepting the painful experiences they have gone through, but that doesn't mean they have dealt with and healed from the impact of the trauma itself. For example, it is possible for a grown child to forgive their narcissistic mother but still struggle with trust issues, insecurities, and identity issues years after the abuse occurred.

Part of recovering from trauma requires understanding the various ways it can impact different aspects of identity. Let's explore some of those areas of impact.

Emotional

Emotional reactions to trauma vary depending on how someone is raised, their unique personality, environmental influences, and the amount of support they have at home or a community level. There are no right or wrong emotional reactions to trauma since survivors choose how to perceive and make sense of their life-threatening circumstances. Common emotions that surface for many people are fear, anger, shame, loneliness, and sadness.

Some survivors do not show emotions, but that doesn't mean they don't feel anything. Often, when emotional expression is not encouraged in the social setting (e.g., a child being ridiculed for crying), the emotions are hidden. Survivors eventually disconnect from their emotions and later on have trouble identifying and processing their unresolved emotions (e.g., an adult who struggles to control their anger because they suppressed it as a teenager).

Physical

A lot of emphasis is placed on the psychological impact of trauma, and not much focus is spent on the physiological symptoms of trauma. When trauma is trapped in the body, it seeks a way out through physical symptoms of poor health. These might include symptoms like unexpected migraines, stomach problems, hypertension, heart palpitations, skin disorders, respiratory disorders, sleep disturbances, and substance use disorders.

A biological explanation for this is that trauma activates the body's stress response to prepare the survivor for fight-flight-freeze modes. The stress response is not supposed to be turned on for an extended period because all of the adrenaline and stress hormones put a severe strain on other vital organs in the body. Subsequently, unresolved trauma that is stored in the body for months and years weakens the immune system, which lowers the defense against infections and diseases.

Cognitive

Trauma affects both the brain and the psychological mind. On a neurological level, trauma impacts the ability to learn, concentrate, memorize information, make rational choices, and regulate emotions. A common sign of PTSD is having cognitive distortions, which are thinking errors that are created by misinterpreting experiences that resemble the previous trauma as threatening.

Survivors may also attempt to make sense of their past traumas by assuming an unreasonable amount of responsibility and carrying unjustified guilt. If the perpetrator was a parental figure, they might idealize them and attempt to rationalize their harmful behaviors. Another way that trauma affects thinking patterns and behaviors is by creating intrusive thoughts and memories that emerge without warning. If undetected, they can trigger strong emotional reactions. When intrusive thoughts and memories occur, they can retraumatize survivors and reinforce trauma-based responses, ultimately making it challenging to heal.

Behavioral

Trauma activates the fight, flight, and freeze responses. This means that survivors can react to trauma in different ways, namely by showing signs of aggressive behavior, physically or emotionally distancing themselves, or becoming avoidant and detached from the situation. The behavioral reactions to trauma also depend on what kinds of coping mechanisms survivors have adopted.

For example, someone might cope with ongoing symptoms of PTSD by working excessively, while another person might cope by developing gambling or overspending habits. Other behavioral signs of trauma are compulsive or impulsive behaviors like overeating (or starving yourself), binging on food and alcohol (as well as emotional eating), and high-risk behaviors like having multiple sex partners or incurring debt on a credit card.

Social

Going through a traumatic experience or multiple experiences compromises survivors' sense of safety and community. More often than not, it is the people closest to them, their relatives, romantic partners, or friends, who are the perpetrators. Survivors may isolate themselves from others completely or depend excessively on others to cope with the stress in the aftermath of the trauma. This can lead to unhealthy relationship dynamics that cause codependency, narcissism, and manipulation.

The stigma around mental health and trauma makes it difficult for survivors to seek help or confide in their close network of friends and family. It is common for survivors, more especially men, to suppress their trauma symptoms and develop alternative obsessions to distract themselves, such as work, physical exercise, promiscuous lifestyle, or addictive substances. When trauma is related to a breakdown of trust, survivors may avoid forming close and intimate relationships with others, which protects them from getting hurt but also prevents them from fulfilling their need for connection.

Developmental

Young children and older people are at a higher risk of developing trauma due to their vulnerability to stress. Unlike other age groups, they have fewer options available to protect themselves against perceived threats. Nevertheless, symptoms of trauma are seen in people of all ages, genders, sexual orientations, religions, and cultural and ethnic backgrounds. In other words, the identity of an individual does not make them immune to traumatic experiences.

In a report titled *Trauma-Informed Care in Behavioral Health Services* by the Substance Abuse and Mental Health Services Administration (SAMHSA), a real-life case study about a young lady named Sadhanna is shared that illustrates the effects of the factors mentioned above (SAMHSA, 2014). Sadhanna is a 22-year-old female who was mandated by the court to outpatient substance abuse and mental health treatment as an alternative to going to prison. Sadhanna was arrested and appeared before the court for assaulting a woman on the street. She admitted that the whole incident was a blur because she was intoxicated at the time the assault took place.

For seven years, Sadhanna struggled with alcohol abuse and had a depressive episode at 18. She also reported being physically abused by her mother's boyfriend from the age of 4 until she was 15. What surprised mental health workers was Sadhanna's emotionless narration of her traumatic past. She showed signs of being detached not only from her feelings and experiences but also from the treatment process. She told a staff member that she didn't want to attend group therapy and listen to people talk about their feelings because she had learned a long time ago never to show emotions (SAMHSA, 2014).

How to Identify Traumatic Shadows

You may be someone who can acknowledge and identify the trauma wounds from your past. Alternatively, you may acknowledge living with unresolved trauma but struggle to identify what wounds you are carrying and from which particular life experiences they originate. If you resonate with the latter, you may be experiencing traumatic shadows; these are signs and symptoms that point to your underlying wounds but disguise themselves as normal behavioral reactions.

What makes traumatic shadows tough to identify is that they don't feel like they have anything to do with your past traumatic experiences. Moreover, the fact that most people in society are stressed and burned out nowadays makes it harder to associate your symptoms with past trauma. In other words, not every stress symptom you feel is necessarily due to your demanding job, lack of sleep, or difficult relationships. Some symptoms can be linked to PTSD responses.

The following list outlines the common signs and symptoms of trauma:

- poor concentration
- depression
- hopelessness
- irritability
- flashbacks
- nightmares
- anger issues
- crying spells
- unjustified guilt

- unexplained exhaustion
- loss of motivation
- difficulty sleeping
- loss of sex drive
- difficulty trusting people
- avoiding things related to trauma
- seeing danger everywhere
- feeling jittery and on guard
- feeling inferior or inadequate

Identifying your traumatic shadows is the first step to uncovering the deeper trauma wound that is hidden in your unconscious mind. Once you have acknowledged the signs of trauma, you can go deeper and explore your symptoms using the following steps.

Step 1: Acknowledge the Pain

Spend time by yourself reflecting on your life. Tune in to your mind and body and observe what thoughts and emotions come to the surface. Hold space for your emotions without judging their appropriateness. Whisper to yourself, "What hurts right now? What feels off? What am I denying?"

Think about your general state of mind and health over the years and the life situations you have been through. Consider how small day-to-day crises or recent life changes have created pain. Perhaps you have normalized the pain to the extent that it feels normal to carry the hurt. Or maybe you are continuously exposed to the source of your triggers, which makes it difficult to address the pain. Now is your time to bring those minor and major hurts to the surface and acknowledge them.

Step 2: Show Curiosity

Lean into the pain and get curious. Challenge yourself to maintain an open heart as you embrace the emotional discomfort. The aim is to get as close to the core wound as possible, which requires you to be willing to explore your emotions. For example, pain is the blanket emotion that covers raw emotions like betrayal, shame, anger, humiliation, fear, abandonment, and rejection.

To figure out which raw emotions are behind your pain, recall a time in your childhood when you presented an emotional need to your parents or caregivers and were shut down. How did you react to their dismissal of your need? Here are some of the ways children respond in similar situations:

- crying
- going silent
- withdrawing
- behaving differently
- throwing a tantrum
- caring less about things
- trying to win parents' approval

Being shut down consistently caused you to believe that your needs didn't matter and, therefore, didn't deserve to be communicated. This thought is painful because it forces you to rethink who you are and how you ought to relate to others. Eventually, you might assume that since your needs don't matter, you don't matter either. Moreover, as a child, you are more likely to blame yourself for the shortcomings of your parents or caregivers. For instance, if you are given silent treatment by a parent, you may feel guilty for provoking them to behave in that manner.

Raw emotions like shame, fear, anger, rejection, and abandonment can be traced back to these early childhood memories of being denied certain needs and making interpretations about what that meant for you. The trauma wound is caused by feeling emotionally neglected, vulnerable, and insecure. You were hurting, and nobody noticed. You needed help, but nobody cared. You showed excitement but were mocked. You displayed vulnerability and got punished. These experiences are extremely painful for people at any age, particularly children who are still finding themselves and need guidance and nurturing from their parents.

Step 3: Connect the Dots

Go back to the beginning and look over your traumatic shadows, the signs and symptoms of trauma that became part of your daily experiences. Make a connection between your symptoms and the trauma wound you are carrying. Examine whether these symptoms appeared when you were a child or adolescent or if they were once coping mechanisms that you turned to.

For example, were you an irritable child or teenager who isolated yourself often? Did you have sleep disturbances and unexplained migraines? The PTSD symptoms that you experienced back then could have become "normal" health conditions later in life. Alternatively, if you were a child or teenager who suppressed your emotions and masked your symptoms with good behaviors (e.g., being a top-achiever at school), you may reach a stage in adulthood where you can no longer contain the pain. Every thought, emotion, or impulse that you denied may come exploding out of you through:

- erratic and irrational behaviors
- mental burnout
- extreme risk-taking
- perfectionism
- uncontrollable anger
- avoidance of people
- defensive attitudes
- excessive criticism and judgment of self and others

Connecting the dots is about acknowledging the golden thread between your traumatic shadows (i.e., trauma-informed behaviors) and the deeper trauma wound that is buried in your unconscious mind.

Embarking on Your Trauma Recovery Journey With Shadow Work

Trauma is energy that is stored in the body as unprocessed pain. The pain is pushed down into the unconscious mind, where it cannot be felt or detected. Nevertheless, the pain resurfaces without notice whenever the trauma wound is triggered. This is usually when you act out of character and do things you normally wouldn't do. The purpose of shadow work is to bring up and push out this energy so that you can heal the trauma wound and reconcile your thoughts and feelings about the past.

To bring up unprocessed pain, you must be willing to feel it. Through practices like meditation, mindfulness, and journaling, shadow work encourages you to engage with your memories and traumas and work through difficult emotions. Feeling the pain and responding with acceptance and compassion enable you to transform your relationship with your emotions. Instead of continuing the cycle of numbing, avoiding, or denying unpleasant emotions, you can allow them to surface, make their presence known, and naturally subside or flow out of you.

To remain open and curious as you bring up and push out unprocessed pain, you must feel safe. Thus, shadow work helps you regain a sense of personal safety (i.e., safety exploring your thoughts and feelings) by promoting nonjudgmental awareness and self-compassion. Trauma shatters your safety bubble and sometimes causes a collapse of your belief systems or sense of right and wrong. Before you can trust others again, you need to completely trust yourself. Getting to a place where you can embrace vulnerability without feeling threatened takes practice and patience. However, the ongoing commitment to connect with deeper aspects of yourself can give you the courage to accept and express who you are and not feel afraid to do so.

Trauma isn't something that you can just "get over" with time. The energy that has been trapped in your body for all these years needs to go somewhere. Shadow work not only brings your attention to unresolved trauma, but it can also give you a healthy outlet to process the pain and return to a whole and undivided self. To feel your pain you need to be tuned in to your mind and body and feel safe connecting to your thoughts, beliefs, emotions, and memories.

The shadow work process guides you through this journey of regaining a sense of safety in your body and nurturing yourself back to health.

Additional Help and Resources for Trauma Survivors

Learning more about your trauma can make the process of addressing your wounds feel less intimidating. The reason why you are living with trauma is because, at some stage in your life, you experienced or witnessed physical or emotional pain and abuse. The harm may have been inflicted on you or the people around you. Depending on how you were impacted by the threatening event or series of events, you developed one of the following types of trauma:

- acute trauma resulting from a single distressing event (e.g., getting involved in a car accident)

- chronic trauma resulting from ongoing exposure to distressful events (e.g., childhood emotional neglect)

- complex trauma resulting from multiple and varied types of distressing events (e.g., sexual abuse, domestic violence, and bullying)

- secondary trauma resulting from witnessing someone within close contact experience a distressing event or ongoing trauma (e.g., witnessing parents' physically abusive relationship)

Recovering from trauma occurs in stages that can spread over years. The day you decide to finally confront your trauma is not the same day you completely heal. Therefore, it is important to manage your expectations when embarking on the trauma-healing journey to ensure you stay focused and motivated at every stage.

The five stages of trauma recovery are as follows (Swaim, 2022):

- **Stage 1: pre-trauma characteristics:** During this stage, you are unaware of your trauma or PTSD symptoms and continue living your life as usual. You maintain the same mindset, attitudes, and behaviors that constitute the norm.

- **Stage 2: rumination:** Something in your life shifts and creates an opportunity for you to question how you are living. This leads to challenging your current beliefs and behaviors and being curious about the impact of your past. You may experience intrusive thoughts and memories at this stage.

- **Stage 3: event centrality:** In this stage, you can identify and reflect on your trauma and make a connection to how it has affected different areas of your life. You may also feel a strong desire to process your trauma and heal. At this stage, you are willing to make the necessary cognitive and psychosocial changes to improve your life.

- **Stage 4: control:** This stage involves taking action on healing trauma by seeking help, going on a treatment plan, and practicing therapeutic techniques like shadow work. Moreover, during this stage, you get to assess the effectiveness of your coping mechanisms and adopt healthier ones that can help you with self-regulation.

- **Stage 5: mastery:** Over time, you will begin to see the positive results of healing trauma. There may be some uncomfortable adjustments you have to make, like adopting healthier habits and routines, but these changes significantly improve your quality of life. Furthermore, you may still experience trauma symptoms like intrusive thoughts; however, they no longer have control over your mental and emotional state.

Please note that your trauma healing journey may look slightly different from these stages, which is normal. What's important is to ensure that you are making progress, no matter how small or different it may look. The following tips are essential to remember when recovering from trauma:

- **Healing is not a competition.** Avoid the temptation to measure your healing journey with somebody else's. You may have gone through similar experiences, but how you have been impacted by your trauma or how you mentally and emotionally make sense of your trauma will be different.

- **Bring your whole self to the process.** Take into consideration the various components of self that influence how you respond to trauma. Think about the impact of your age, gender, race, religion, ethnicity, and cultural background on how you make sense of your trauma.

- **Realize that post-traumatic growth can happen.** We often talk about PTSD and overlook the growth that can take place post-trauma. Examples of post-traumatic growth include personal development, greater appreciation for life, discovering a sense of purpose, and improving the quality of your relationships.

• **Be willing to accept support.** Your recovery doesn't need to be experienced in isolation. Reach out to your support system and share with them the journey you are on. Let them know how they can assist you with practical everyday errands or emotional support. Help may also come from therapists, support groups, and forums where others are on the same journey as you.

• **Avoid recreational substances.** Mind-altering drugs or substances are not recommended during recovery since they can affect your moods, thought processes, and behaviors. Some substances like marijuana or alcohol have a numbing effect, which prevents you from working through your feelings.

• **Practice self-care.** It is crucial to listen to your mind and body when recovering from trauma to avoid pushing yourself to the limits. Get into the habit of taking short breaks during the day to check on yourself and respond to your needs. Make time for yourself in the mornings or evenings to reflect, relax, and creatively express how you are feeling.

Recovery from trauma requires an investment of your time and effort. However, the journey doesn't need to be a lonely one. There are resources and virtual communities available to support you through the recovery process. You may also benefit from starting individual or group therapy. Some of the most effective therapies for treating trauma include cognitive behavioral therapy (CBT), dialectical behavioral therapy (DBT), trauma-informed therapy, prolonged exposure therapy, and eye movement desensitization and reprocessing therapy (EMDR).

For emergency assistance, don't hesitate to reach out to the U.S. crisis hotlines listed below (APA, 2021):

• National Alliance on Mental Illness: (800) 950-NAMI(6264)

• National Sexual Assault Hotline: (800)-656-HOPE(4673)

• National Suicide and Crisis Lifeline: 988

• LGBTQ National Hotline: (888) 843-4564

• Substance Abuse and Mental Health Services Administration: 1-800-662-HELP (4357)

Shadow Work Journal Prompts

1. What was the hardest day you experienced as a child? Describe the events that took place.

2. Recall a time when you felt unheard by your parents or caregivers. How did you react?

3. When you feel unheard as an adult, how do you normally react? How similar or different is this to how you responded to being unheard as a child?

4. What were the unspoken rules in your family household? Make a list.

5. How did these unspoken rules affect your ability to share your honest thoughts and feelings?

6. What family secrets were you forced to keep? How has being burdened with secrets affected your adult life?

7. Identify a fear that can be traced back to early childhood trauma. Suggest ways that you can overcome this fear.

8. Describe your family dynamics growing up. How did these relational patterns affect how you build relationships with other people today?

9. What were the money beliefs you were taught as a child? How have these beliefs influenced how you manage finances?

10. How was the concept of love modeled by your parents? How do you express love to others today?

11. Describe a harmful coping mechanism that you developed as a child that continues to complicate your life or relationships today.

12. Is there somebody from your childhood that you feared? Why did you fear them? How do you relate with people who have similar personalities today?

13. Think back to a time in the past when you felt completely safe and trusting. How can you recreate that experience in your life now?

**14. What does support mean to you?
What types of support do you need from others?**

15. What childhood dreams were abandoned due to the interruption of trauma? How can you revive and explore those dreams today?

16. What life lessons have you learned from your childhood upbringing? How can you incorporate those lessons in the way you live?

17. Write a letter to a younger version of yourself who felt helpless.
In the letter, show empathy for his or her situation
and offer encouraging words they can hold onto.

18. Has your childhood trauma affected your sense of self-worth?
If so, write down practical daily practices that you can do to boost
your confidence and embrace your inherent worth.

19. Identify someone who played the role of a mentor growing up. Write a thank you letter to them to express your gratitude for their support (you do not have to send the letter to them).

20. Did your childhood upbringing negatively impact your educational prospects? If so, how can you invest in your education now? What online resources or formal courses can you take to accelerate your personal growth?

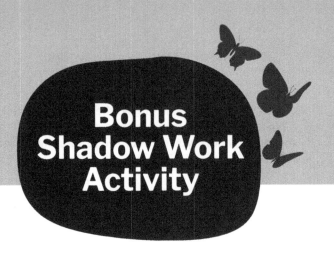

Bonus Shadow Work Activity

Trauma Breathwork Activity

Breathwork is the practice of conscious breathing that helps you regulate your nervous system, reduce stress, and manage acute and chronic pain. Trauma breathwork deals specifically with processing and releasing trauma trapped in the body. It works by putting you in a deep state of relaxation where you can bypass your conscious mind and create space for unconscious thoughts, emotions, or impulses to come up during the session. As the sensations surface, they are released through intentional breathing, one breath at a time.

Trauma breathwork counters the body's stress response by deactivating the fight-flight-freeze mode. This means that you have the freedom to connect to deep emotions and process them without losing control of your body. The process promotes emotional healing and acceptance and leaves you feeling lighter and grounded at the end.

Dutch endurance athlete Wim Hof developed a breathwork exercise known as the Wim Hof Method, which reduces stress, boosts the immune system, and enhances performance (Nash, 2023). The Wim Hof Method is effective for controlling emotional triggers, impulsivity, or chronic stress. Practicing this method consistently can improve your stress tolerance levels and help you cope with symptoms of PTSD.

Instructions (Othership, 2021):

1. Sit or lay down in a comfortable position with your eyes closed.

2. Breathe through your nose and out of your mouth. Feel your stomach rise and collapse with every inhale and exhale.

3.   Take 30–40 deep breaths (in through the nose and out through the mouth) without any breaks in between the inhalation and exhalation. Do not be alarmed if you feel lightheaded; it is a normal sensation to feel during this step.

4.   On your 30th or 40th exhale, take a deep breath and hold it for as long as you can (maximum one minute). Exhale slowly out of your mouth.

5.   On your next inhale, hold your breath for 15 seconds, then breathe out slowly.

6.   Repeat this sequence 3–4 times without pausing.

Experiencing symptoms of trauma is an invitation to dig up and process trauma wounds that have been stored in your unconscious mind. Through shadow work, you can identify trauma-based responses, trace where they originate, and heal the root cause of your trauma. In the following chapter, we will explore what happens after trauma wounds have been processed and released, which is another process known as shadow integration.

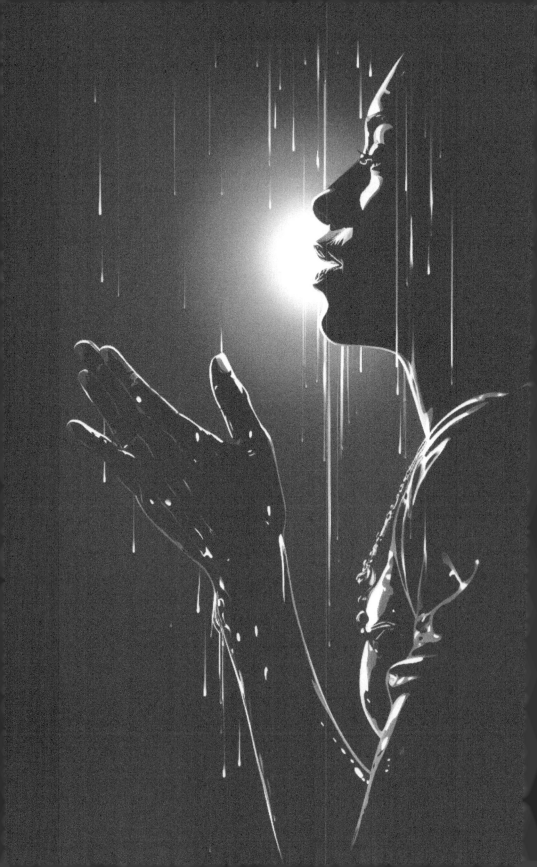

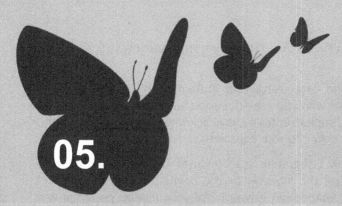

05.

Integrating Your Shadow for a Whole You

If you don't accept yourself, you can't transcend yourself and the world: first, you need to increase your awareness, then you need to accept what you learn, then you need to take action. –Oli Anderson

Why You Should Integrate Your Shadow

We have discussed the importance of uprooting trauma from your unconscious mind and processing it through shadow work. However, the healing journey doesn't end there. Once you have unearthed and processed your trauma, the next and most important step is to reclaim your fragmented selves.

After experiencing a traumatic event, your whole identity splits into different "selves." We touched on these two selves earlier in Chapter 1 when looking at how the shadow self manifests. The identity split creates a conscious and unconscious self: the "you" that you are aware of and the "you" that you are blindsided by. Part of your healing journey is to not only address your traumas and emotional issues but also to reintegrate these two selves to restore your whole identity. In a nutshell, this is what shadow integration is all about.

The word *integrate* comes from the Latin root word *integer*, which means whole. Therefore, to integrate something is to put together separate parts of something, or someone, and make a whole object.

Being authentic and expressing your authentic self requires you to accept every part of who you are—the good and the ugly—and reclaim them. You are not complete until you have acknowledged, embraced, and integrated your shadow into your conscious personality.

The goal of shadow integration is to uncover the repressed aspects of yourself, including the inner gold—the positive traits, desires, and dreams that were abandoned in youth. All your hidden potential and shortcomings, the strengths and weaknesses, are brought to the surface and reconstructed into your identity. You will no longer have different personas or social masks that you wear whenever it is convenient for you. Your only persona will be your true self, the unapologetic, self-aware, and empowered version of yourself.

There are several benefits to practicing shadow integration, such as

- **supporting personal growth and development:** Shadow integration helps you work through the mental barriers and emotional issues that are standing in the way of your greatness. The process challenges you to step outside of your comfort zone, confront old cycles and patterns, and rediscover who you are.

- **learning more about yourself:** There are aspects of your character and personal history that you have denied or forgotten. Shadow integration lifts the unconscious veil and exposes these parts of you. This isn't done to shame you but rather to cultivate self-awareness and enable you to see yourself from an objective view.

- **identifying triggers and past traumas:** Shadow integration helps you travel deep into your unconscious mind and locate the root cause of your triggers and traumas. Exposing the wounds can bring healing but also create an opportunity to gain insights and life lessons from the pain.

Shadow integration is a powerful process that can help people who are dealing with all sorts of physical or psychological issues. For example, those who are struggling with addiction or impulsive behaviors can use shadow integration to understand the motivation behind their urges or cravings. People who suffer from periodic aches and pains can use shadow integration to track the cycles and patterns of their pain and connect this with emotional wounds that may be triggered. People who are going through a difficult life transition or those who may be feeling stuck or overwhelmed can use shadow integration to gain a sense of direction, enhance self-acceptance, and transform their lives.

How to Practice Shadow Integration

Carl Jung believed that self-actualization was possible through achieving wholeness, not perfection. A whole individual isn't somebody without sin, but instead, somebody who acknowledges and accepts their sinful nature and integrates it with other "good" elements of their identity.

Shadow integration challenges you to develop a new relationship with your shadow, one where you are capable of seeing the potential in your darkness. You are called to see the opportunity for conquering your deepest fears, overcoming your insecurities, and parenting your wounded inner child who cries out for the needs they were robbed of in childhood. Even though your shadow has the capacity for destruction, shadow integration allows you to learn from your pain and use it as a resource to develop a more robust character.

What good can come out of my aggression? you might wonder. To see the potential good that can come from your aggression, start by exploring the emotion deeper. Travel back in time and recall the earliest memories of feeling angry. Consider what motivated you to choose this particular emotional reaction. What did you want to achieve? What did you secretly desire? Perhaps being aggressive was a way to distract your parents from fighting with each other. What you secretly desired was inner and outer peace. Or maybe your anger was a way to get attention from your preoccupied parents. In those moments, you desired affection and reassurance.

Through shadow integration, you can transform your aggression into the purest desire or motivation that exists behind it. However, to do this, you must be willing to accept your aggression and understand how it has assisted you throughout these years. Certainly, it isn't the healthiest coping mechanism, but over the years, it has enabled you to express needs that you were too afraid to boldly come out and ask for. When you have come to terms with your aggression and no longer need to hide behind it, you can connect to your deeper needs and motivations (i.e., inner peace, affection, seeking reassurance) and find positive ways to address them.

The following steps provide a framework for practicing shadow integration. How you choose to practice shadow integration may slightly deviate from the framework. The purpose of giving you this outline is to show you how to unearth repressed emotions and transform them into a desired experience.

Step 1: Spend Time in Silence

To connect to your shadow, you must break through the conscious barriers of your mind. This is possible when you can spend time in silent meditation and quiet your mind. If many thoughts are racing through your mind, practice noticing without unpacking them. It is normal to feel bored when you are spending time in silence. However, boredom doesn't have to be seen as a bad thing. Boredom can be a gateway to reflecting on your mental and emotional well-being, an opportunity to check in with yourself. Avoid the temptation to fill your silence with activities or distractions. Sit quietly, close your eyes, and allow your body to rest.

Step 2: Invite the Darkness

Now that you are relaxed and your mind is open, you have the liberty to travel to the past and bring up a distressing emotion that you have a difficult time accepting. It may be easier to recall the earliest situation where the emotion was triggered. Be prepared to feel uncomfortable and have a set of coping skills ready to practice when an unpleasant emotion emerges.

Create a mental picture of what the emotion looks like. Is it a person that you recognize? A fictional character? A monstrous animal? An innocent child? Or an overwhelming force of nature (e.g., wind, fire). Make the image crystal clear in your mind, as if you were standing in front of the emotion. Notice how you feel looking at it. Are you scared? Sad? Disappointed? You can also notice the thoughts that come to your mind as you acknowledge the emotion. Do you hear words spoken by your parents? What is your inner critic saying? Are the thoughts intensifying your emotion?

Step 3: Observe Without Attachment

It is normal to feel strong resistance at this stage. Everything inside of you will be pushing toward a reaction. You will be tempted to handle the emotion in the same way you have always handled it. Nevertheless, remind yourself that you are not your emotions. You are the observer of your emotions. Therefore, you are not attached to your emotions, even though you have compassion for how you are feeling. Be aware of your role as observer, the one who is doing the watching. Your awareness is like the expansive blue sky, and your emotions are the clouds passing by.

Step 4: Track the Origin

At this stage, you have created enough distance between yourself and the emotion to examine it completely. With a curious mind, investigate where and when the emotion originated. Go back to the specific date, time, and location when you felt the emotion (if you can remember). Reflect on the situation that was taking place. For example, who was there? What was the occasion? Was there any dialogue, if so, what was said? How did the situation unfold and eventually end? Determine when and how your emotion developed. What specifically triggered it? What sensations went through your body? What thoughts were going through your mind?

Step 5: Allow the Emotion to Move Through You

Up until this point, you have been observing the unpleasant emotion. Permit yourself now to embody the emotion by getting inside your younger self's body. Feel the emotion as strongly as you felt it back then. Let it move through your body and become what it wants to be. If you feel the urge to cry, yell, or scream, don't hold back. If there are words you would like to express, let them out. If you feel like running or dancing, feel free to do so. You are not expected to show any restraint in how you express the emotion, except for not harming yourself or others.

Finally, speak to the emotion and share how it has brought you discomfort for all the years. Explain how reacting this way has compromised aspects of your life. Describe the negative ripple effect on your health, habits, and relationships. Thank your emotion for giving you a voice when you didn't have one and for protecting you in its way. Express your desire to heal and learn how to address your needs directly without hiding behind your emotions. Feel a sense of peace as you let go of attaching yourself to the emotion. Return to your role as observer and look over your emotion with compassion. Notice the shift of energy as you move from attachment to observation.

Step 6: Be Honest About What You Want

During this final stage, you get to choose what you want. Go back to the situation that triggered your strong emotion. Connect to that little boy or little girl's heart and determine what he or she needed at that moment that couldn't be expressed in words. Was it respect? Nurturing? Acceptance? From now onward, you can make a conscious choice to respond to the unmet need behind the emotion whenever you are triggered or resort to the same explosive emotional reaction. The fact that you can see both choices means that you have successfully integrated an aspect of your shadow into your conscious identity. Neither choice is more powerful than the other. As the observer, who is not particularly attached to any choice, you can make a decision that is in your best interest.

Shadow Integration Tips

Shadow integration can be challenging due to the intense emotional journey you are taking on, but this doesn't make it impossible. The following tips will make the shadow integration process easier and more enriching:

- **Center yourself.** Get into a calm, clear, and neutral state of mind before you start the process. Postpone the session if you are having a bad day or have a lot on your mind. Use breathwork to calm your mind and body and prepare you for the journey.

- **Show compassion.** Confronting aspects of the shadow is uncomfortable. Ease yourself into the process by being gentle and compassionate toward yourself. Let go of judgments and adopt a curious and understanding attitude. Reassure yourself that you are safe and nothing bad will happen to you.

- **Have a reflective mindset.** Be willing to reflect on your thoughts, emotions, and reactions without criticism. Constantly ask yourself "why" to go deeper into your unconscious mind. Approach shadow integration with the aim of walking away having learned something new about yourself.

- **Be honest with yourself.** Be willing to tell the truth about what you are thinking and feeling. Remember that you are not going to be judged or punished for what you discover. Moreover, accept the full range of your emotions and be courageous enough to sit with your feelings, even the difficult ones. When you feel the resistance getting stronger, see this as a sign that you are getting closer to the source of pain.

- **Document your discoveries.** During or after the process, write down notes about your experience. Think about what stood out for you and any breakthroughs you were able to achieve. If there are any themes you would like to delve deeper into in your journaling sessions, write these down too.

One of the challenges you may experience when performing shadow integration is the inability to detach from your self-identity. Instead of seeing yourself as one-dimensional, choose to see yourself as being multidimensional. The self-image that you have developed over the years is only one aspect of a larger identity. The other deeper parts of yourself can be discovered by observing your mind and being open to learning new things about yourself.

How Journaling Helps With Shadow Integration

In the first chapter, you were introduced to shadow work journaling, a therapeutic technique that enables you to examine your shadow and bring up the repressed parts of your personality for healing purposes. The same method is helpful during shadow integration to identify and process unpleasant memories, thoughts, and feelings that are behind your triggers, negative patterns, and impulsive behaviors.

It is not always obvious why you behave the way you do or how some emotions you experience are deeply entrenched in your past. Shadow work journaling helps you understand yourself better and the underlying motivations behind your actions and reactions. The benefits of practicing shadow work journaling for shadow integration are

- teaching you how to identify the shadow and bring wounds to the surface,
- helping you connect the dots between your thoughts, emotions, and behaviors,
- creating a more systematic approach to shadow work so that you can track your progress,
- getting the opportunity to cultivate self-awareness and develop a stronger relationship with yourself,
- encouraging you to form healthier relationships with others,
- developing emotional resilience to manage difficult moments, and
- helping you to embrace vulnerability and be honest about your thoughts and emotions.

When using shadow journaling for shadow integration, there are simple steps to follow that can enhance your experience.

Step 1: Find a Quiet Place

Find a corner or room at home where you can spend time journaling without any interruptions. Since the process can be emotional, it is recommended to find an area where you feel safe and comfortable.

Step 2: Pick a Topic

Decide on a topic you would like to explore. This could be a recurring theme in your life, a troubling childhood memory, a distressing emotion, or an unhealthy habit that you would like to investigate.

If you don't have a topic, you can start writing and see what thoughts spontaneously come to your mind. Alternatively, you can have a dialogue with your shadow (i.e., going back and forth, switching between yourself and your shadow) or use a list of journal prompts to assist you.

Step 3: Start the Clock and Write

Set a timer for 5–10 minutes, depending on how much time you have to spare. If you can write for longer, you can increase the timer to 15–30 minutes. As you write, you are welcome to add drawings, symbols, or keywords that appear in your mind and help you express yourself more authentically.

Step 4: Dig Deeper

The most crucial step is to challenge and question why certain things have occurred or continue to happen in your life. There are four steps that you can follow to ensure that your journaling practice is impactful and achieves the goals of shadow integration.

Diagnose the Issue

Be clear on what issue you are going to explore during the session. Focus on a single issue to avoid complicating the process. These questions will help you get to the core issue you are seeking to resolve:

- In what area are you struggling?
- What hurts?
- What unhealthy patterns keep occurring?

Link the Issue With the Emotional Reaction

You need to understand how your everyday issues are associated with your emotional reactions. Your emotions are the gateway to unresolved trauma, limiting beliefs, and other emotional issues. These questions will help you link the issue with your emotions:

- How does this struggle make you feel?
- How do you feel when a certain thing hurts?
- What intense emotions trigger the pattern?

Connecting the Dots

Once you have identified the core emotions, connect them to the earliest memories you have of experiencing them. If you cannot remember that far back, think of the most recent time you have felt the emotion. These questions will help you create the connection:

- Can you recall the first time you felt this emotion?

- How has the emotion appeared throughout your life?

- If this emotion is associated with an unmet need, can you recall the first experience of not having your need met?

Pave the Way Forward

Now that you can start to see the light, shift your focus to what you desire in place of the emotion. Consider the possibilities of healing the emotion and adopting positive coping mechanisms. These questions will help you clarify the way forward:

- How would you like to feel most of the time?

- How do you want to feel about a specific triggering situation?

- What unmet need can you address instead of overreacting?

Step 5: Review

After going through the journaling exercise, stand back and review what you were able to come up with. Remember to review previous journal entries as well to make sense of where you are along your journey. As you read the entries, notice new and emerging patterns of your thoughts, emotions, and motivations.

Shadow work journaling exposes the raw and hidden parts of you. Use the coping strategies provided earlier in this book to manage strong emotions. Moreover, choose to see the inner resistance or emotional blocks as opportunities to lean into the process, not step away. For best results, establish a consistent journaling routine and take action on your discoveries.

Shadow Work Journal Prompts

1. What situations make you feel most vulnerable? Why?

2. What qualities do you admire in others but cannot trace in yourself?

3. What emotions are you afraid of embracing? Why?

4. Do you often get intrusive thoughts? What are they?

5. What aspects of your physical appearance are you ashamed of?

6. What aspects of your personality are you ashamed of?

7. Do you often change your persona in front of different people? Why?

8. What things about your past does your inner critic often remind you about?

9. What experiences have you convinced yourself you can live without?

10. What things do you normally lie about, even if they are white lies?

11. In which social contexts do you find yourself "trying too hard?" Why?

12. In which social contexts do you find yourself taking a backseat? Why?

13. What emotional experience takes place inside of you when being criticized?

14.Do you dream or frequently have nightmares? What do they mean to you?

15. In what ways do you self-sabotage? Describe three scenarios.

16. When you are feeling defensive, how do you behave? Identify five defensive behaviors you often display.

17. Who do you still seek validation from, even if you are ashamed to admit it?

18. "I am a difficult person to love."
Explore this statement and explain what it means to you.

19. Which parts of your childhood are painful to revisit? Why?

20. If you could turn back time and relive a memory from childhood, which would it be?

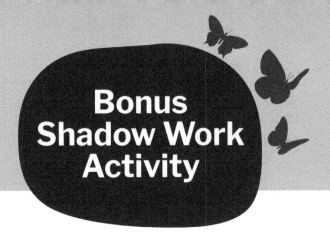

Bonus Shadow Work Activity

Shadow Work Affirmations

You may be familiar with positive affirmations. These are positive statements, written in the present tense, which reinforce new patterns of thinking and feeling. Shadow work affirmations are similar in that they help to rewire your thought processes and positively change how you perceive your life. During the final step of shadow integration, where you have the freedom to choose what you want, shadow work affirmations can assist in forming and reinforcing new patterns of thoughts, emotions, and behaviors that you desire.

With that said, shadow work affirmations are not always positive. Some affirmations have negative words that are used to positively shift your perception of yourself and your life circumstances. You may also find uplifting affirmations and intense affirmations, but combined, they can help you integrate your shadow with your conscious identity and feel balanced and grounded.

Here are 30 shadow work affirmations to assist with shadow integration:

1. I choose growth over comfort.
2. I am capable of healing.
3. I am not defined by my past.
4. I am proud of who I am.
5. My thoughts and emotions matter.
6. My happiness is my own responsibility.
7. I deserve to receive love as effortlessly as I show love.
8. My problems present growth opportunities.
9. I welcome change and new experiences.
10. I let go of holding grudges and practice forgiveness.
11. My life is as important as everyone else's.

12. It is my responsibility to protect my inner child.
13. It is not my fault that people behave the way they do.
14. I am stronger for sitting with my uncomfortable feelings.
15. I am grateful for the life lessons taught by my struggles.
16. In every situation, I have a choice on how to respond.
17. I am not responsible for how people perceive me.
18. Dealing with pain is not an excuse to treat others poorly.
19. I accept my mistakes but choose not to define myself by them.
20. I accept that my parents did the best they could to raise me.
21. I am making peace with my shadow to avoid hurting others.
22. I am grateful for painful experiences that taught me compassion.
23. I have the choice to let go of negativity when it no longer serves me.
24. Relationships that take more energy than they give back are not for me.
25. I let go of seeking love from people who are incapable of showing it.
26. Forgiveness is a gateway to healing myself. I deserve to be at peace.
27. I let go of seeking approval from others. I choose to celebrate myself.
28. Everything that happens in my life teaches me the value and power of love.
29. I invite relationships that uplift me. I stay away from relationships that drain me.
30. I am not responsible for the suffering in my childhood, but I am responsible for healing from it.

Shadow integration is about reconciling your split identity to create a whole and authentic identity that embraces every aspect of who you are. The process is intense but achievable through honesty, self-compassion, and willingness to uncover the deeper parts of yourself.

We have now completed the second part of the book, where we discussed how shadow work can support your trauma recovery and shadow integration journeys. You have been equipped with the necessary tools and skills to proceed to the third part of the book, which takes you through the transformative benefits of shadow work.

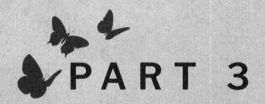

PART 3

UNDERSTANDING
SHADOW WORK

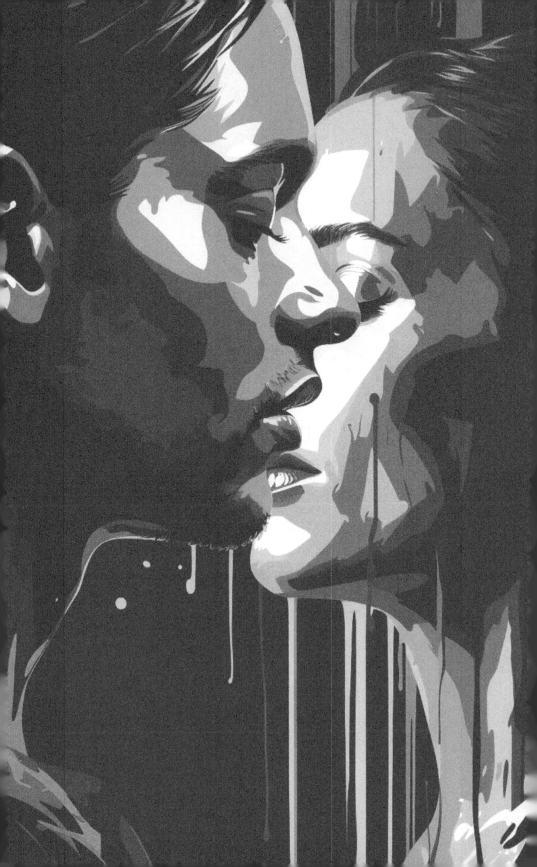

Enhancing Your Relationships Through Shadow Work

The shadow is a moral problem that challenges the whole ego-personality, for no one can become conscious of the shadow without considerable moral effort. Becoming conscious of it involves recognizing the dark aspects of the personality as present and real.
–Carl Jung

Psychological Projection in Relationships

One of the ways that your ego defends itself is through a process known as psychological projection, which refers to misdirecting your difficult emotions, impulses, and negative attributes on someone else rather than acknowledging and accepting them as your own.

Your ego cannot tolerate being wrong, receiving criticism, feeling inferior to others, and any other unpleasant emotion that would destabilize your constructed self-image. Therefore, to avoid dealing with your dark traits or confronting your shortcomings, your ego projects those qualities it deems unacceptable or inappropriate to others.

Psychological projections are so powerful that you are often unaware they are occurring. In the heat of the moment, when your triggers are activated, your instinctual reaction is to defend yourself at all costs. Furthermore, your conscious mind has a list of reasons to justify your need to say hurtful words or misbehave.

Projections feel safe because they protect you from awakening your trauma wounds and having to confront the fears and insecurities you have shoved deep inside your unconscious mind.

Nonetheless, continuing to support your projections can compromise the quality of your relationships since you are not engaging with what is happening in the present moment but, instead, reacting from a deep place of hurt. Moreover, the inability to accept every aspect of yourself and love yourself unconditionally makes it harder for you to extend warmth, acceptance, and compassion toward others. In other words, psychological projections create emotional blocks inside of you that get in the way of truly seeing people for who they are and being able to connect and build safe and nurturing relationships.

Here's an example of how projection works:

Julian was raised by a narcissistic mother. His coping mechanism as a child was to withdraw and suppress his emotions. Throughout his adult life, he has had difficult relationships with women that are connected to his dysfunctional relationship with his mother. Julian projects his feelings of anger and mistrust for his mother onto his romantic partners. His ex-girlfriends describe him as a bully, controlling, and jealous. He shows blatant disrespect for women because he lost respect for his mother as a child. He struggles to form a deep and nourishing emotional bond beyond sexual intimacy because he was robbed of the emotional connection with his mother.

Over time, psychological projection caused Julian to become the image of what he feared the most. Julian developed narcissistic traits due to not addressing the wounds of being raised by a narcissistic mother. He may not even be aware of how similar his toxic behaviors are to the trauma he experienced as a child. If someone points out his behaviors, Julian is more likely to attack that person (ego defense mechanism) instead of processing and reflecting on what has been said and doing shadow work to see whether their feedback is valid or not.

Psychological projections can also have a positive aspect, whereby you see the potential or greatness of others that you fail to recognize or cultivate inside yourself. Think about the ways people react to celebrities or anyone they admire. They put them on pedestals and assign them positive attributes that the celebrities may or may not possess. Idolizing celebrities is a way for them to escape embodying their greatness. Perhaps due to harboring insecurities or being afraid of failure, they are not willing to tap into the golden aspects of their shadows.

Whether you are projecting the qualities that you like or dislike, the fact remains that your relationships suffer when you run away from confronting your shadow. Shadow work teaches you to pay attention to your state of mind and take responsibility for how you may be feeling and how you are impacted by others' behaviors. It shows you how to recognize defensive behavior and when you might be triggered by what others have said or done. Moreover, shadow work helps you crack through the defense mechanism of the ego, so you can address the agonizing emotional pain that interferes with building healthy relationships with others.

How Shadow Work Improves Your Relationships

We have discussed how shadow work assists with trauma recovery and shadow integration; however, shadow work can also improve your platonic, romantic, and professional relationships. Relationships can be challenging to navigate because of the unique individuals that come together to build them. Even though you may have things in common with your loved ones, you may have different childhood upbringings, trauma wounds, life experiences, mindsets and beliefs, and so on.

The personal history and baggage that both you and your loved ones bring into your relationships create conflicting ideas about how your relationships are supposed to be managed and what roles or expectations each person is supposed to fulfill. Added to this, the unresolved traumas and emotional issues from past relationships can cause conflict and misunderstandings.

Shadow work strengthens relationships by strengthening the individuals inside of them. The process promotes self-awareness and self-exploration, which are fundamental tools for getting to know yourself better and identifying unconscious patterns that are triggered in your relationships. By acknowledging your dark side, including the destructive behaviors that can sabotage your relationships, you can overcome the barriers to intimacy and connection.

The type of love that we call toxic is the manifestation of unhealed shadows in relationships. This toxic love can be seen between parents and children, best friends, or romantic partners. Due to one or both parties' unwillingness to address their traumas, insecurities, irrational fears, or relationship issues (e.g., trust issues, commitment issues, intimacy issues), they project these unacknowledged wounds onto their loved ones. The result is ongoing conflict, dysfunctional relationship dynamics, and resentment. Consider the following examples of how the shadow impacts loving relationships:

- A mother obsessed with her children's safety may have control issues.

- A romantic partner with an abandonment wound may be needy or possessive.

- A friend who has a rejection wound may have codependency issues.

- A sibling who has body image issues may struggle with feelings of envy.

- A father who was abused as a child may suffer from substance abuse problems.

- A romantic partner who was sexually abused may avoid sexual intimacy.

Shadow Work and Romance

One of the ways to practice shadow work is to embark on the journey with your romantic partner. The health of your romantic relationship requires juggling the needs of four entities: you, your partner, and both of your shadows. You and your partner may have spent a lot of time getting to know each other, but if your shadows cannot relate to and understand each other, they can clash and cause irreparable damage.

Practicing shadow work as a couple can be a powerful way to cultivate emotional intimacy and connect on a deeper level. Instead of accepting each other at face value, you can learn the patterns that inform how both of you think, feel, and behave. Furthermore, you have a unique opportunity to hold space for each other and be a mirror, taking turns to uncover blindspots, confront weaknesses, and come face-to-face with your fears. The frameworks used to practice shadow work are the same for couples as they are for individuals. The only difference is that you have someone to hold you accountable and provide loving support throughout the process. Consider having a shadow work journal that you share as a couple where you can complete relationship journal prompts and discuss your entries.

Singles who are looking for love can also benefit from practicing shadow work during the searching stage. Think of it as a way to confront and heal from your emotional baggage before stepping into your next relationship. Of course, the healing journey is continuous, and you will need to practice shadow work once you do enter a relationship. However, getting a head start and clearing as many unconscious beliefs and emotions as you can will increase your chances of attracting healthy partners who are also on their journey of healing and personal growth.

Another opportune time to practice shadow work is after a breakup. No matter how cordial the breakup is, it can trigger old wounds, fears, negative beliefs, and impulsive behaviors. You may feel guilty, angry, rejected, or disorientated by the sudden split or toxic cycle that has finally come to an end. Shadow work can help you manage your dark side and avoid the common unhelpful reactions of passing blame, projecting your feelings, or seeking revenge.

Acknowledging and calming down your shadow can take some time, especially when the relationship is tumultuous, and a trauma bond has been created. However, when the storm has finally cleared, and you are ready to accept the good and bad aspects of the relationship, you can take an honest look at yourself and identify patterns that may have led to the breakup and what you can do differently in your next relationship.

Become an Effective Communicator With Shadow Work

Effective communication is about listening to understand where someone is coming from and connecting to the intention behind their message—this form of communication challenges you to focus on understanding rather than seeking to be understood. When you focus attentively on the message someone is conveying, the conversation becomes less about your needs or opinions. They receive your undivided attention, and you can respond from a place of empathy instead of defensiveness.

Shadow work cultivates self-awareness and helps you learn how to become an effective communicator. Through reflections and journaling, you can assess the quality of your interactions with others and identify communication barriers that make it difficult for others to openly express their thoughts and feelings to you (or personal hangups that make it difficult to convey your thoughts and feelings to others). Typical challenges that cause communication problems are

- **stress and feeling emotionally overwhelmed:** When your stress response is activated, your main focus is addressing survival needs. During this state, you may be more selfish than usual and struggle to pause and listen to others. Additionally, stress can make you highly sensitive to perceived threats, which means that you are more likely to misinterpret what others are saying or overreact to minor situations.

- **conflict and misunderstandings:** Back-and-forth arguing or making accusations to win arguments won't help you reach resolutions. Listening is an essential component of effective communication. Without it, you can't put yourself in another person's shoes and understand where they are coming from. Withholding judgments during conflict and maintaining an open mind can lower your defenses and help you focus on the message conveyed.

- **lack of focus:** It is impossible to fully grasp what someone is saying when you are distracted. Signs of a lack of focus include multitasking, looking away when someone is speaking, scrolling through your phone, or daydreaming. Effective communication requires you to extract the meaning from the information shared with you. To do this, you need to be paying attention to both verbal and nonverbal cues.

How often do you think about your reply or formulate a counterargument while someone is speaking? You might grab onto the first three words or sentences and then take a mental shortcut and assume you know which direction they are heading. The risk of taking the mental shortcut is that you might misunderstand the intent behind their message. Think about the times when your sincere questions or comments were twisted and made out to be something they weren't.

The secret to being an effective communicator is to approach conversations with mindfulness. As mentioned earlier, mindfulness is the practice of being present in the moment and embracing the experiences that are emerging. Mindful communication challenges you to enter conversations without assumptions. Imagine that whatever you are going to hear will be heard for the first time. There is no history or background to base your opinions on. The only way to understand the speaker is to listen to every word coming out of their mouth, notice the tone and language they are using, observe their body language, and look for any other clues that can help you draw factual conclusions.

Mindful communication considers what others are thinking and feeling in the moment but also how you might be positively or negatively impacting their ability to share their thoughts and feelings. In other words, you are conscious of the power or influence you might carry that can affect how the conversation progresses. A manager who is conscious of their authoritative position will pay attention to how they approach conversations with their employees, realizing the difficulty their employees might have in freely sharing their thoughts. To make them feel comfortable opening up, the manager might have an open door policy, encourage ideas and feedback, show interest in their team's personal lives, and validate their team's concerns to make them feel seen.

Mindful communication has many benefits, such as cultivating self-awareness, strengthening relationships, and improving your mental health. Research has shown that mindful communicators show emotional resilience and can regulate their moods during stressful times (Blain, 2023). Having greater self-control and awareness makes you less likely to project your thoughts and feelings onto others. Moreover, you are capable of resolving conflict without blowing the situation out of proportion.

There are a few tips that you can practice to become mindful when communicating with others:

• **Learn to forgive and see the good in others.** Forgiving others is not easy, and neither is practicing gratitude. However, these traits can positively transform your thinking patterns and help you display emotional control during conversations. Challenge yourself to forgive three people each day and write down three things that you appreciate about them.

• **Be compassionate with yourself and others.** Go into conversations without carrying expectations of how the interaction will go or what you need the other person to say or do. Adapt to their moods and attitudes without taking offense. Imagine what they may be experiencing on an unconscious level. When you are having a bad day, be extra sensitive to your needs. Remind yourself that everyone has shadow moments sometimes.

• **Be willing to offer an apology.** Don't wait to be asked for an apology. When you notice the unintended negative impact you have made on someone, say sorry. Those simple words validate how they might be feeling and enable reconciliation to take place. If you have more power and influence, offering an apology makes the less powerful person feel seen.

• **Be conscientious.** Pay attention to your body language, facial expressions, tone of voice, and the presence you carry into a room. Remember that people are not only impacted by your words but also by the way you present yourself. Seek feedback from a few close people to get a better understanding of how others perceive you. This can help you make the necessary adjustments to make a positive impression on others.

• **Create healthy boundaries.** Being mindful isn't the same as being a pushover. Learn how to separate your thoughts and emotions from the way other people think and feel so that you can set healthy limits that protect you from being disrespected, exploited, or manipulated. For example, you may be willing to listen to an angry friend express their frustration with you, but you interject or disengage the moment they start yelling.

The tips mentioned here apply to all types of relationships, both personal and professional.

How to Cultivate Empathy With Shadow Work

The ability to have honest and meaningful interactions with others rests on your capacity to show empathy toward them. This is easier to do when you are on the same page and share common ideas and perspectives. However, when you argue or feel strongly against their behaviors, showing empathy becomes harder.

Empathy has nothing to do with agreement. You don't need to accept or support a loved one's actions to empathize with them. To show empathy means to see the world from the other person's viewpoint and imagine what they are thinking or feeling. The purpose of this is to understand where they are coming from and what informs their decisions or behaviors. At the end of the exercise, you may still hold firmly to your opinions about the matter, but at least you have an idea of how where the clash between you lies.

Cultivating empathy can significantly improve your shadow work. Many of the traumas and emotional issues you are carrying have to do with someone or multiple people who failed you in the past. Part of unpacking and processing these wounds requires exploring what motivated those people to behave the way they did. What were they thinking or feeling at the time? Why did they hurt you? Without practicing empathy, it will be difficult for you to immerse yourself in their reality and see life from their perspective. You won't be able to connect to their thought processes and understand their behaviors.

Here's an example of empathy in action during shadow work:

Cassie recently broke up with her boyfriend of two years. The couple met at a mutual friend's barbecue and instantly fell in love with each other. Their relationship was going steady for the first year, and the pair was beginning to make plans for marriage. However, a sudden downsizing at her boyfriend's place of work left him without a job. He remained optimistic during the first few months of unemployment and submitted his résumé to every nearby company with vacancies. But with every rejection notice, his confidence was taking a knock.

Her boyfriend's attitude changed toward her when he had used up the money in his savings and couldn't financially contribute to their household bills. He began talking down to her, starting small fights, withholding intimacy, and developing new habits like staying out late with his friends. The relationship took a turn for the worse when Cassie learned about her boyfriend's infidelity. That was her breaking point. As much as she loved him and was willing to support him during this rough patch in his life, she had to walk away.

For months after the breakup, Cassie was furious at her ex-boyfriend for how the relationship turned out. She blamed him for placing his needs above the relationship. Cassie decided to practice shadow work as part of her recovery from the breakup. She wanted to understand how her unconscious beliefs and behaviors could have contributed to the collapse of her relationship and what could have motivated her ex-boyfriend to cheat.

She discovered that money was a central theme in their relationship. Her love language was gift-buying, and she placed a lot of value on the lifestyle that her ex-boyfriend provided. He, on the other hand, held traditional masculine values of being a protector and provider and felt validated and respected when he could take care of their household. The relationship was going steady because there was financial stability, but when her ex-boyfriend lost the means to provide, his shadow was triggered, and the relationship suffered.

Cassie understood that for her ex-boyfriend, being able to provide made him feel worthy as a man. Due to his upbringing and social conditioning, his sense of self-worth was strongly connected to his level of competence. Being unemployed made him feel like an inferior man who was unworthy of receiving love from his woman. The cheating was a byproduct of his low self-esteem, negative self-talk, and self-sabotaging behaviors that ultimately turned him into someone Cassie couldn't recognize. After empathizing with her ex-boyfriend, Cassie was able to move on from the relationship and continue working on her healing journey.

If you are interested in incorporating empathy into your shadow work, follow these simple guidelines:

- **Embrace differences.** Learn not to expect others to think or feel the same way you do. Be open to the various beliefs and motivations other people use to navigate their lives. Consider how being raised in different racial, cultural, or social backgrounds plays a role in how someone views the world. Embrace the idea that there are multiple ways to experience a common situation.

- **Identify common ground.** Even though you are different from the next person, you share universal human experiences like feeling pain or desiring peace. Step away from your differences and search for common ground. What can you both agree on? What needs, fears, or desires do you share?

- **Ask open-ended questions.** When you ask questions, you open the space to learn from the other person. It can also prevent you from making quick judgments based on what you perceive is happening. Use questions to clarify your assumptions, understand the other person's thought processes, and learn more about their perspectives.

- **Understand your empathy blocks.** Everybody has empathy blocks, those topics or experiences where they find it difficult to connect and relate with others. Use shadow work meditation or journaling to identify your empathy blocks and trace where they come from and how they affect your ability to connect and relate. Practice overcoming the inner resistance that these blocks cause through shadow integration.

- **Second-guess yourself.** Be willing to be wrong about someone in hopes that you may walk away having learned something new about them. Empathy tests your level of openness to people and experiences that fall outside your realm of comfort. The more you step into the unknown, the less information you will have to support your ideas. Allow the interactions you have with people to expand your mind and challenge your existing beliefs.

These tips apply to all types of relationships, both personal and professional.

Shadow Work Journal Prompts

1. What kind of behaviors performed by other people trigger you?
   Reflect on how this could be a psychological projection.

2. How does your childhood relationship with your parents affect how you
   navigate adult relationships?

3. What type of people do you find difficult to tolerate? How do they resemble people from your past?

4. What relationship boundaries were violated as a child? How do you reinforce those boundaries in your current relationships?

5. What are your core relationship values?
Why are these values important to you?

6. Define what trust means to you.
How has trust been honored or dishonored in your relationships?

7. Identify three shadow traits that frequently show up in your relationships. What are the needs or motivations behind these traits?

8. Recall a time when someone gave you feedback that you struggled to accept. What thoughts and emotions did you feel? How did you perceive the situation?

9. Describe your relationship with sensuality and sexual intimacy. What do these terms mean for you? What challenges have you faced embracing your sensuality and sexuality in the past?

10. How important is it for you to feel a sense of power and control in a relationship? Why?

11. What role do you usually play in romantic relationships? How is this role informed by your history and social conditioning?

12. Describe your relationship with forgiveness and some of the breakthroughs and challenges you have experienced in the past.

13. Which current relationships are you grateful for?
How do these relationships impact your life?

14. What do masculinity and femininity mean to you?
Which of these energies do you resonate with, and why?

15. Reflect on your family dynamics. Which family members are you close with and estranged from? What would you change?

16. Reflect on a time when you felt betrayed as a child. Who betrayed you? What were your unspoken expectations for that individual? What needs were unfulfilled?

17. Describe your relationship with your career. How was the concept of work introduced to you? What is the significance of working?

18. Would you describe yourself as someone who is emotionally expressive? What struggles do you encounter when sharing your honest thoughts and emotions (if any)?

19. What is the purpose of your relationships? Reflect on the purpose of your friendships, family bonds, and romantic relationships (or ones you aspire to have).

20. How comfortable are you with change in relationships? How can you create space for your loved ones to grow without compromising your relationships with them?

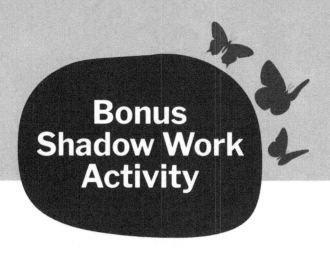

Bonus Shadow Work Activity

3-2-1 Shadow Process

Philosopher Ken Wilber is known for a famous technique he invented to approach shadow integration, known as the 3-2-1 process (Hussain, 2020). The technique encourages you to identify psychological projections directed toward people (or their behaviors) and understand the deeper meaning behind them.

The first step is to imagine you are looking at the person who has triggered you from a third-person perspective (e.g., What are they doing?). Second, imagine yourself confronting them by asking a question or expressing what you dislike. This allows you to take on a second-person perspective (e.g., "Why do you behave that way?). Finally, imagine yourself becoming that person and stepping into their reality. Empathize with their behavior from a first-person perspective (e.g., I behave this way because...).

By the time you have switched to all three perspectives, the hope is that you will be able to look at the triggering behavior from an objective view and acknowledge how you may have been reacting to your fears, assumptions, or defensiveness.

Shadow work shows you how the greatest enemy is the one within, not the one outside. By practicing mindful communication and empathy and being aware of your projections, you can learn to accept and be more understanding toward your loved ones. In the next chapter, we will take a look at ways to respond to common challenges during shadow work.

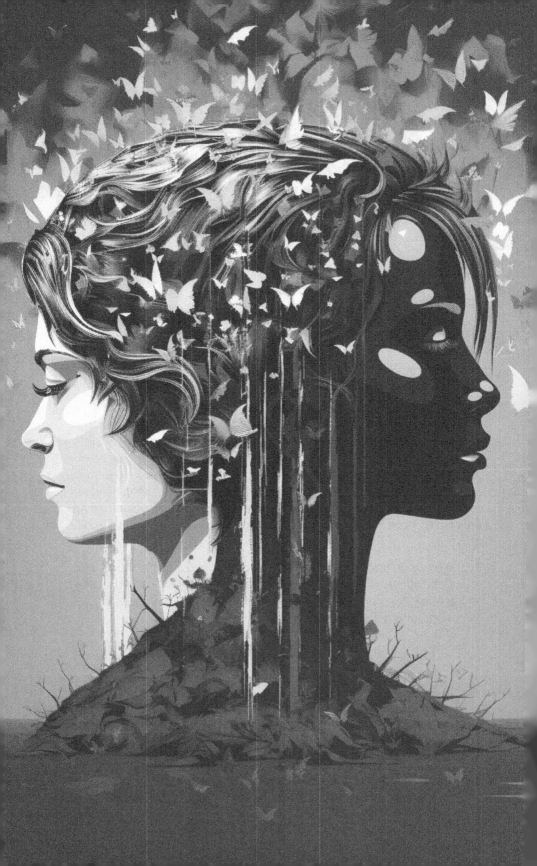

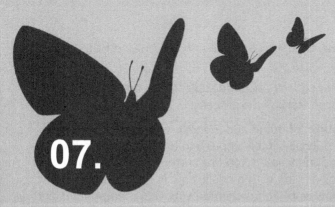

07.

Overcoming Common Shadow Work Challenges

People are afraid of shadows. People are even more afraid of being in the shadow. But without a shadow, life will be two-dimensional.

–Yoko Ono

Challenges Are Normal in the Shadow Work Process

When you hit roadblocks during shadow work, don't take it as a sign to quit or doubt yourself. Challenges are part of the process of uncovering your shadow and addressing your emotional issues. They are proof that you have lifted the veil of the conscious self and are entering depths of your mind that haven't been explored before.

We can liken the experience of shadow work to the process of disinfecting an open physical wound. Is the process dangerous? Certainly not. However, it is profoundly uncomfortable and frustrating. Nevertheless, when you have gone through the agony of removing the bacteria from the open wound, you can bandage the area and allow it to slowly close and heal. Shadow work is the painful cost you pay to address trauma from the past. After you have sat through the discomfort, you can lovingly step away from the wound and give it time to heal.

To make the experience less uncomfortable, there are a few ways to prepare yourself before starting the process:

- **Check your state of mind.** Be honest with yourself—are you mentally and emotionally stable enough to explore your shadow and dig up painful experiences? If you are currently overwhelmed with responsibilities or dealing with a crisis, now is not the best time to commence shadow work. Focus on improving your mental health and regaining a sense of calm and order before you start.

- **Anticipate change.** One thing is for sure, your life will not be the same on the other side of shadow work. Mentally prepare yourself for the shift in your thoughts, beliefs, and habits. Realize that when you learn new information about who you are, you will feel a strong desire to outgrow your current lifestyle. Adopt a positive outlook on change. Choose to see what you gain rather than what you might lose.

- **Prepare for the highs and lows.** The emotional regulation skills taught earlier in the book will help you cope with waves of unpleasant emotions, inner resistance, and the fear of vulnerability. Use these skills, along with the stress management techniques outlined in the following sections, to manage the fluctuations in your moods and any emotional blocks you may experience.

- **Find the right support.** Identify a few people who you can reach out to when the process gets tough, and you need some encouragement. These could be people you live with, like your spouse or sibling, or professional mental health providers who can create a supportive environment for you to engage with your inner world. You can also look for support groups online that provide peer support or coaching on how to go through each step of shadow work.

- **Balance shadow work with self-care.** Give yourself breaks during shadow work to respond to your needs and allow your mind and body to rest. Incorporate self-care practices into your daily routine that promote stress management, relaxation, creativity, and connecting with others. If you are someone who feels guilty for practicing self-care, investigate why that is through shadow work journaling. Remind yourself that you matter, and be intentional about scheduling time to nurture yourself.

How to Overcome Setbacks and Frustrations

Shadow work compels you to confront your darkest fears, and that can be intimidating. Setbacks occur because the process itself is incredibly challenging and not because you aren't putting in enough effort. Nevertheless, this doesn't prevent feelings of disappointment every time you fail to achieve a desired milestone.

Before embarking on shadow work, take the time to redefine how you view setbacks so that you find it easy to bounce back after encountering one. Like many people, you may view setbacks as evidence of failure and personal inadequacy. As a result, you may feel less enthusiastic about pursuing your goals after several failed attempts. But there is another way of viewing setbacks that allows you to see them as a part of the learning process, not the end of a journey.

Challenge yourself to start thinking of setbacks as intentional errors that reveal your blindspots and help you sharpen your focus. Without these errors, you wouldn't have the room to grow or master your skills. Setbacks help you take a step back, reflect on your actions, and determine what you may be unconsciously doing to compromise your results. Redefining setbacks in this way motivates you to take back control of your journey. Since shadow work can be strenuous, your ability to regain control and immediately get back on track helps you sustain a positive attitude during the highs and lows.

Furthermore, there are coping skills that you can practice whenever you experience setbacks that make getting back up easier:

- **Look for the lesson.** Put a positive twist on failure by searching for the lesson. Reflect on the lessons you can take from the experience. How did you grow from it? How did your strategies improve from then?

- **Take an alternative path.** Learning from setbacks means being willing to adapt to the situation and find other ways to reach your goals. For example, if your third attempt at shadow work meditation fails, see it as an opportunity to explore alternative shadow work practices that can achieve the same outcomes. Don't feel rushed to choose an alternative path either. Take a break from the process and go back to the drawing board.

- **Challenge negative thoughts.** Criticizing yourself after setbacks is a counterintuitive coping mechanism that prolongs your suffering and keeps you down permanently. To uplift yourself, you need to keep your thoughts positive through practices like shadow work affirmations. Whenever negative thoughts emerge, take a moment to pause and acknowledge that you have derailed your desired thinking pattern. Adjust the negative thought so that it is fair and balanced (i.e., not black or white, jumping to the worst conclusions).

Frustration is the feeling of irritation at not being able to change or achieve a desired result. Setbacks come with a lot of frustration because they make you aware of a barrier that you cannot overcome. The positive side of feeling frustrated is that you can identify that something to do with the process isn't working as planned; however, when you dwell on the emotion of frustration too long, you lose sight of the real problem and get wrapped up in the feeling.

To avoid being distracted by the frustration that comes with setbacks, try the following stress management techniques to calm your nervous system and activate your rational mind:

- meditate
- say a prayer
- practice breathwork
- complete a workout
- spend time outdoors
- practice journaling
- listen to music
- practice self-care
- find a positive distraction

Frustration is also related to anger. Thus, if you notice something deeper triggering your frustration besides the temporary setback, spend time investigating what that might be. For example, your frustration may be rooted in your childhood, where you were compared to your siblings, struggled at school, or experienced developmental challenges that made it hard for you to learn behaviors as quickly as other children. Bring up the repressed anger you may be harboring from the past and learn to sit with it, talk to it, and respond to the underlying need (e.g., support, inclusion, acceptance, patience).

Tips for Facing Unpleasant Truths

Like any form of psychotherapy, shadow work brings you face-to-face with the truth about your life. This may come as a shock to you, particularly when you are not yet prepared to burst your bubble of disillusionment. The aim of revealing the truth is not to shame you but rather to bring you to a place of self-acceptance where you are completely transparent and comfortable with yourself.

It takes courage to face the truth about your life because what you learn may not always be pleasant or support the ideas and beliefs you uphold about yourself. For example, you may describe yourself as a confident person but, through shadow work, discover that you are plagued with insecurities. The so-called confidence you believed you had was people-pleasing, a coping mechanism learned during childhood.

The truth sometimes challenges your constructed self-image and perceptions of reality. The ego self doesn't like this at all because everything you had based your life on up until this point could cease to exist. There is a metaphoric death that occurs when you face unpleasant truths about your life—the death of your defenses, the death of your ignorance, the death of your victimhood, and so on. Superficial aspects of yourself that were built to protect you from pain and trauma dissolve, making room for your authentic self to emerge.

Facing the truth requires you to be willing to admit that you don't know everything about yourself and dare to seek answers. Next are some tips on how you can overcome the discomfort around discovering and accepting the truth.

See Reality for What It Is

Acknowledging the truth means being willing to see reality for what it is, not what you desire it to be. Of course, doing this isn't easy because you need to let go of your fantasies, assumptions, or expectations and accept what is presented to you right now. Nevertheless, there is freedom in this because you can release the burden of stress, worry, and disappointment and learn to be content with your current life circumstances or commence the healing process.

Embrace Your Emotions

The other side of accepting your truth is establishing a healthy relationship with your emotions, especially the difficult ones. You are encouraged to be honest and transparent about how you are feeling—first to yourself and then to others. Resist the urge to label your feelings as "good" and "bad," as doing this can cause you to reject unpleasant emotions. Instead, see your emotions as the body's messengers that help you navigate different life situations and learn more about yourself.

Share the Truth With Someone

You need to hear yourself speaking the truth to validate your experiences. Identify someone you trust and feel safe with to open up to about your thoughts and feelings. Approach this individual whenever you need to vent or work through difficult emotions. They don't need to give you advice or feedback. They simply need to hold space while you share what is on your mind. If you cannot find someone within your immediate circle, look for a counselor, coach, or support group.

Commit to Take Action

What happens after you have discovered the truth? You take action and bring about the necessary changes in your life. Complete healing and recovery isn't possible until you have "cleaned the wound." Thus, use the insights or information you have learned to start implementing changes. There are times when taking action is not applicable. For example, you might learn the truth about your childhood, but you cannot go back and change what happened. Or you might learn the truth behind your loved one's destructive behaviors, but you cannot change who they are as a person.

When taking action isn't possible, consider how you can avoid repeating the same patterns or mistakes in the future. For example, how can you be a better parent for your children to ensure they don't succumb to the same traumas you experienced as a child? Or how can you be more intentional about building healthy relationships to avoid attracting negative people in your life?

As challenging as it may be to face the truth, you have what it takes. Remind yourself regularly of the benefits of acknowledging and speaking your truth. Imagine the ways it can positively enrich your life and relationships.

Working Through Fears

Is there a part of you that is scared to confront your truth or uncover aspects of yourself that have been transferred to your shadow? If so, understand that this feeling is normal. Fear is a natural response whenever you venture outside of your realm of safety. A reasonable amount of fear is good because it shows that you are pushing the boundaries of your mind. However, too much fear can be paralyzing and get in the way of fully engaging in the shadow work process.

One of the most effective ways to work through your fears is to name them. Describe what exactly you are afraid of and put a face to it. This can help you take an abstract emotion and confine it to something very specific. For example, instead of being afraid of shadow work because you don't know what to expect, go deeper and figure out which elements of the process frighten you. Label your fears and understand what beliefs are fueling them.

For example, you might discover that your fear of shadow work centers around the need for vulnerability. Perhaps reflecting and acknowledging your trauma is something you find easy because it requires tapping into your mind. However, processing, embracing, and empathizing with your trauma could be something you find difficult because it requires opening your heart. Having discovered the root of your fear, you have more knowledge of your strengths and weaknesses going into shadow work and specific areas that require more attention and compassion.

You will notice that you have more control over your fears when you can list what they are, how they impact you, where they come from, and when they are triggered. They may not disappear after all of this, but at least you can anticipate them and plan effective coping skills to practice when they arise. There are other helpful tips that you can practice to work through your fears, such as

- **Talk to yourself about your fears.** Have an open and honest dialogue with yourself about your fears. Switch between your ego self (i.e., identity that protects your fears) and your wise self (i.e., identity that overcomes your fears) and ask questions about what you are afraid of or what might happen if you confront your fears. Continue to talk to yourself until you feel less anxious about overcoming your fears.

- **Develop trust in yourself.** Once again, consider how much personal power you have given over to your fears. Imagine how different your attitude would be if you reinvested all of that power into cultivating self-confidence and fortifying your mind. Remember that while you cannot control external outcomes, you can influence them by controlling your thoughts, emotions, and motivations. Place more trust in yourself than in the process because you have the power to influence how the process turns out.

- **Focus on your desired results.** Be intentional about where you place your energy. If you focus all of your energy on the fear itself, it is magnified and becomes a wall that you find difficult to climb over. However, when you focus on the desired results, you are motivated to apply your mind to think of solutions to address potential setbacks.

• **Don't rest your identity on the outcomes.** Resist the urge to base thoughts and feelings about yourself on your shadow work progress. For example, do not think "I will be proud of myself if I complete this process" or "My happiness depends on reaching this milestone." This mentality puts a lot of pressure on you to prove yourself right to maintain a positive self-image. Moreover, failing to achieve the desired results can impact your self-worth.

You have the inner knowledge to overcome your fears. The challenge, however, is learning to redirect your focus to your skills and competencies rather than on your fears. The more time you spend empowering yourself, the smaller your fears become in comparison to you.

How to Handle Feelings of Overwhelm

Despite how much you attempt to regulate your emotions and go through each step of the shadow work process in record-breaking time, you will have days where you feel overwhelmed. Don't take this as a sign that you haven't mastered your emotions or that perhaps there are aspects of your shadow that you haven't fully accepted. Feeling overwhelmed is a natural human response to stress.

Nothing is alarming about overthinking, saying words you don't mean, being moody, or not having the energy to practice shadow work. No matter how much healing you undertake, you cannot escape the normal and inevitable stressors of life. The reason you may feel overwhelmed is because life is challenging, and some days you don't feel like putting up a fight. What's important is not preventing feelings of overwhelm but having a plan on how to respond when these feelings occur.

Consider the following practical three-step action plan to manage feelings of being overwhelmed.

Notice the Shift or Change

Become so knowledgeable about yourself that you can easily notice sudden shifts in your moods, energy, and behaviors. Learn how to recognize normal thoughts, feelings, and behaviors you display and signs of being overwhelmed. For example, if you are normally a calm and balanced person, having an emotional outburst signals a shift in your demeanor and potentially a sign of something else. Catching these shifts or changes as they happen can make you more aware of your behaviors and provide options for how to self-regulate.

Common signs of being overwhelmed to look out for include

- irrational thoughts
- intrusive thoughts
- feeling like quitting
- feeling restless
- anxiety or panic attacks
- losing motivation
- being pessimistic
- withdrawal from people
- unexplained mood changes
- struggling to make decisions or follow through
- exaggerated emotional or behavioral responses

Investigate

The next step is to find out what caused the sudden shift or change. What might have happened to make you feel overwhelmed? Have there been recent developments in your life that have caught you off guard or added more stress? Could you have been triggered? Investigating your feelings of being overwhelmed prevents you from being stuck on the emotion and struggling to move forward. It can also help you make the necessary adjustments to your life to reduce stress as much as possible.

Here is why you might feel overwhelmed:

- lack of support
- health concerns
- financial concerns
- emotional triggers
- social, economic, or environmental issues
- ongoing conflict in your relationships
- being caught off guard by life-changing events
- taking on too many tasks or responsibilities

Step Forward

Finally, consider what small steps you can take to improve the situation. Don't entertain big decisions like relocating or cutting ties with people. Think small and practical solutions to make you feel better right now. The purpose of making small gestures is to self-soothe and take yourself out of the fight-flight-freeze state. Only then can you start thinking about bigger lifestyle decisions.

The following small and practical activities can help you take a step forward:

- drink a glass of water
- take deep breaths
- play your favorite songs
- look in the mirror and smile
- call a loved one
- take a shower
- take a walk outside
- say a prayer or mantra
- find humor in the situation
- move your body and exercise
- remind yourself of what is within your control
- schedule an appointment with your therapist

Preventing Isolation

Shadow work can sometimes cause you to isolate yourself. This happens for various reasons. For example, you might require privacy or solitude to complete shadow work techniques, or you might have days or weeks of being in a reflective mood and not feeling the desire to interact with people beyond work.

Taking time out for yourself is essential throughout the shadow work process; however, be careful not to use "taking time out" as an excuse to withdraw from everyone. Too much isolation is not a good thing. It can lead to symptoms of loneliness, social anxiety, low self-esteem, and depression. Even when you don't feel like engaging with people, encourage yourself to stay connected to protect your mental health.

Here are the signs your isolation has become unhealthy:

- avoiding social activities and gatherings

- canceling plans with friends and family often

- feeling anxious when thinking about going out

- feeling depressed during periods of solitude

- spending days without contacting anyone

- feeling dread whenever you get a text or call

- feeling emotionally numb or indifferent toward things

There are a few strategies that you can employ to prevent prolonged periods of isolation during shadow work:

- **Practice group self-care.** Find self-care activities that you can do with friends and family, such as sharing a meal, watching a movie, going on a hike, or playing sports.

- **Focus on quality time.** When socializing, be intentional about being in the moment. Avoid distractions like your cell phone or laptop, and give your undivided attention to the person or group of people. After every interaction, reflect on how you feel and what you learned.

- **Find like-minded communities.** Connect with people who share similar values and interests as you or who may also be on their shadow work or trauma recovery journey. Time spent with these people will feel meaningful because you have a lot to talk about and can offer each other the type of social support you are looking for.

- **Know when to seek professional help.** If you notice that you are isolating yourself frequently and have difficulty breaking the pattern, seek the help of a professional who can help you confront and unlearn this behavior as well as identify other underlying mental health conditions like anxiety or depression that may be present.

Shadow Work Journal Prompts

1. What false assumptions do people make about you? In your opinion, why do they perceive you this way?

2. What is a recurring fear that you struggle to combat? What continues to trigger this fear?

3. Think about someone within your close circle (e.g., parents, siblings, best friends). Identify personality traits that you find irritating about this person. Do you share similar traits?

4. Think about someone who hurt you in the past. What are some of the positive life lessons you took from that experience?

5. Describe your relationship with failure. How did you cope with failure as a child? How have your coping mechanisms transformed as an adult?

6. How do you react when you notice being ignored or disregarded? What thoughts fuel this reaction? What is your earliest memory of being ignored or disregarded?

7. Think of somebody whom you don't get along with. Identify three positive attributes about this person.

8. What makes you feel unhappy in romantic relationships? Which of your core needs are overlooked when those behaviors occur?

9. In which areas of your life do you feel underdeveloped or lagging? What would it take to grow in those areas? Who can support you?

10. What does freedom in relationships look like? List some healthy boundaries that can help you achieve this freedom.

11. Define solitude and isolation in your own words.
Reflect on two occasions in your life where you spent time in solitude
and isolation. Describe your emotional experience in both circumstances.

12. Which aspects of shadow work do you find frustrating? Why?

13. Which aspects of shadow work are you afraid of? Why?

14. Recall a situation where you went outside of your comfort zone and felt afraid doing so. Name and describe the fear you felt and how you were able to overcome it.

15. How do you respond to good things happening in your life? Do you celebrate or feel anxious? Do you share the news or pretend like nothing happened? Why do you react this way? Trace your reaction to past experiences.

16. Describe a time when being vulnerable backfired. What limiting beliefs have you carried since that moment? What alternative beliefs can you adopt to improve your relationship with vulnerability? Write them down.

17. What insecurities would people be surprised to learn about you? When did these insecurities develop? How do you mask them?

18. What destructive habit do you want to break? What is the secret pleasure you get from performing this habit? What alternative positive behavior can offer you a similar intensity of pleasure?

19. If your future self sent you a letter describing three important habits to adopt to improve your health, career, and relationships, what would those three habits be?

20. If you could write a letter to your younger self describing the most important realization about life, what realization would that be? How would this information benefit your younger self?

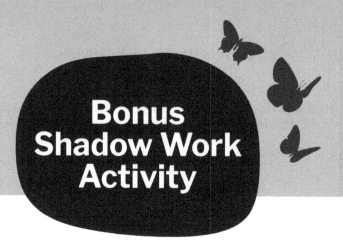

Bonus Shadow Work Activity

Mirror Work

Mirror work is a therapeutic technique developed by motivational coach and author Louise Hay that helps you connect to a deeper part of yourself (Aletheia, 2022). All that you are required to do is stand in front of a mirror for a few minutes and either stare at your reflection or talk to yourself.

As simple as this instruction may sound, mirror work can be challenging. The practice of looking at your reflection can bring up memories, intense emotions, insecurities, or the voice of your inner critic. This happens because the mirror reflects to you what you struggle to accept about yourself. Your openness and willingness to embrace what you metaphorically see in the mirror can promote self-love and self-acceptance.

To add variety to your mirror work sessions, consider the following suggestions:

- recite shadow work affirmations
- speak to your inner child
- identify physical attributes you love
- practice setting boundaries with others
- name and describe how you are feeling
- encourage yourself (practice positive self-talk)

At the end of each session, document your experience and key insights you learned.

Shadow work is challenging but not dangerous or impossible. You may experience setbacks or feel frustrated and fearful along the journey. However, these undesirable lows are part of your process of healing. Learn to expect and embrace them. In the next chapter, we will discuss the importance of celebrating your shadow work victories.

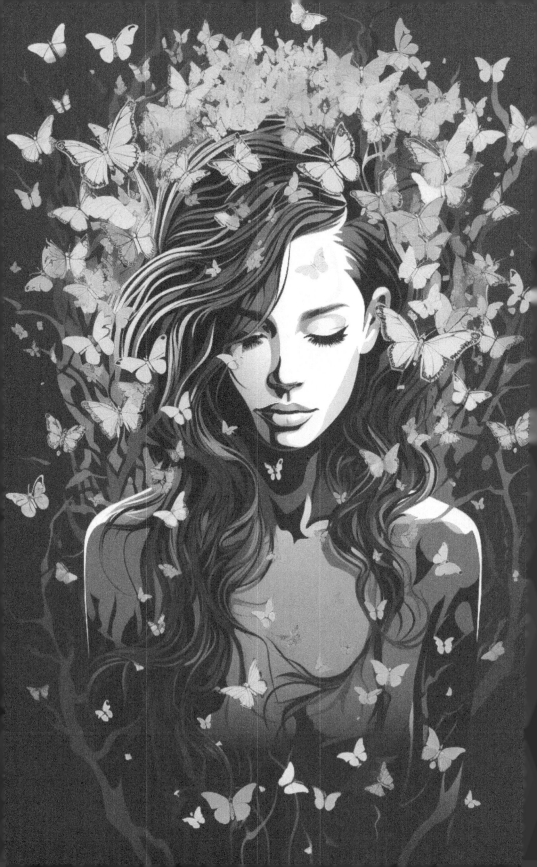

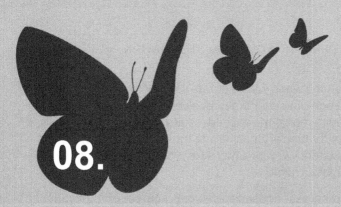

08.

Celebrating Your Transformation

Your life will be transformed when you make peace with your shadow. The caterpillar will become a breathtakingly beautiful butterfly. You will no longer have to pretend to be someone you're not. You will no longer have to prove you're good enough. –Debbie Ford

Celebrating Your Progress

Due to the intense nature of shadow work, it is essential to celebrate your milestones (no matter how small they may be). Granted, you may still have a long way to go before accomplishing your desired results, but the weekly or monthly progress keeps you going. Don't make light of these small transformations. They are proof that the healing process is working.

Celebrating your progress is in itself a practice of gratitude. As Oprah Winfrey once said, "When we celebrate our wins in life, the more we have in life to celebrate" (Lim, 2020). It is a way to remind yourself of how far you have come, what you have been able to achieve, and the exponential growth you have experienced. Without these regular moments of appreciation, the journey toward achieving your goals becomes dull and unmotivating. The weeks and months start looking the same, and you may even lose the drive that got you started in the first place.

The release of dopamine when you celebrate your victories perpetuates the success cycle. Each time your brain receives a reward for a specific action, it is motivated to repeat the desired results to claim more rewards. When there is no celebration after achieving the desired results, there is less urgency or consistency in your actions (i.e., your brain isn't motivated to turn the behavior into a habit).

Celebrating your progress depends on your source of motivation. Generally, there are two types of motivation: intrinsic and extrinsic. Intrinsic motivation refers to the inward-facing desire to succeed. It can be based on your values, beliefs, purpose, or desired state of mind. For example, if you value resilience, take a moment to applaud yourself whenever you successfully manage your emotional triggers. If you desire inner peace and balance, reward yourself each time you prioritize your needs by practicing self-care.

Extrinsic motivation refers to the outward-facing desire to succeed. Here, you are motivated by obtaining symbols of success, such as a healthier lifestyle, job promotions, new relationships, or fresh opportunities. For example, some of your shadow work goals may be based on improving your well-being. Perhaps you want to let go of destructive patterns that cause you to overspend, compromise your health, or get in the way of nurturing your relationships. Every time you make progress on unlearning these patterns (e.g., exercising when you are overwhelmed instead of binging on food), you can take a moment to acknowledge your efforts.

It is important to be creative when choosing the best way to acknowledge and celebrate your progress. Remember, the sweeter the reward, the higher the incentive for your brain to repeat the desired results. Please note that your rewards don't have to cost a lot of money or require extensive planning. They can be simple yet meaningful experiences that make you feel good about the shadow work you are doing.

Here are some suggestions to consider:

- **Make a note of your wins and regularly track your shadow work progress.** Create a log of the milestones you have achieved each week to chart your progress. Decide on a day once a month when you can spend 15 minutes reviewing your progress. Identify things that you did well during the month and decide on an appropriate reward.

- **Pick your top three daily wins.** When setting your intentions for the day, identify three activities that you would like to accomplish by the end of the day to support your shadow work. These should be activities that are realistic and achievable, such as empathizing with your coworkers or recognizing when you are projecting. Have small treats planned for when you accomplish these goals (e.g., listening to your favorite album, or watching an episode of your favorite TV show).

• **Buy a small gift for yourself.** Is there something you have been eyeing in the mall for a while? Wait until you reach a shadow work milestone before you purchase the item. This allows you to make the brain connection between action and reward and motivate yourself to continue the great work. You can also rank the type of gifts you buy based on the size of your milestones. Larger milestones deserve larger gifts.

• **Share the good news with others and allow them to celebrate with you.** It's a good feeling to receive praise for the progress you are making to positively transform your life. Whenever you achieve good results, reach out to a few close friends and family members whom you trust and have confided in before. Share your progress report and thank them for supporting you along the journey.

• **Engage in a bucket list item.** Create a bucket list of activities, hobbies, and experiences you would like to try. These can range from taking creative classes to trying out new restaurants or traveling to a new destination. Whenever you reach a shadow work milestone, refer to your bucket list and choose a relevant item to reward yourself with.

Tips for Making Shadow Work a Lifelong Practice

Throughout the book, you have been shown several ways shadow work can assist with resolving personal life problems and supporting your personal growth. This means that shadow work isn't a one-time endeavor but a continuous practice that you can incorporate into your daily life. How you utilize the techniques of shadow work might change now and again, but the process stays the same.

There are benefits to making shadow work a continuous lifestyle practice, such as

• **Shadow work helps you identify and manage negative emotions.** When you are presented with the inevitable stressors of life, you can use shadow work techniques to regulate your emotions and turn what would have been an explosive reaction or impulsive decision into a controlled response.

CELEBRATING YOUR TRANSFORMATION

- **Shadow work improves your interpersonal relationships.** Shadow work reinforces crucial social skills like empathy, self-awareness, social awareness, and self-regulation. These skills help you communicate your thoughts and feelings effectively, constructively resolve conflict, and be intuitive about the needs of others.

- **Shadow work encourages you to be kind toward yourself.** When you practice shadow work regularly, you learn how to be more accepting of your weaknesses and respond to your pain with self-compassion. Instead of defaulting to judgment, you are challenged to learn from your life experiences and improve each moment.

- **Shadow work promotes good mental health.** If you are prone to stress, shadow work can help you maintain inner peace and balance. When problems arise, you are encouraged to address them immediately using the relevant techniques and modify your behaviors to maintain a sense of emotional control. Shadow work also supports your ongoing treatment for diagnosed mental illnesses, helping you reduce unwanted symptoms like anxiety, mood swings, and overthinking.

- **Shadow work pushes you outside of your comfort zone.** One of the benefits of shadow work is that it challenges you to open your mind and get to know yourself in a way you haven't experienced before. Since there is no limit to your potential, there is no endpoint that you reach during shadow work. In every season of your life, you are exposed to different life challenges that teach you something new about yourself.

- **Shadow work improves emotional resilience.** The techniques practiced during shadow work are created to enhance your self-awareness and self-regulation. This means that over time, you can learn how to anticipate challenging situations and effective ways to manage your emotions and behaviors when they come. Overall, you are given the tools to cope with stress and emotional triggers, so you can make conscious choices about how to respond to situations.

The best way to make shadow work a lifelong practice is to incorporate practices into your daily routine. This requires allocating a minimum of 10 minutes each day or a few times a week to practice shadow work. Identify a time of day when you are least busy. It could be early in the morning before starting your day or late in the evening when you are winding down for bed. Plan which shadow work practices you are going to do, in advance, so that you have the necessary materials when the time arrives.

Here are some beginner-friendly shadow work practices that you can incorporate into your routine.

Shadow Reflection

Discovering your shadow self takes a long time. There are numerous fears, traumas, memories, beliefs, desires, and personality traits that have been transferred to your unconscious mind since childhood. It would take several years to fully grasp your shadow, but by then, your shadow would have evolved, which means the learning is continuous.

Make it a daily practice to reflect on aspects of your shadow. This is an exercise that can be done on the spot. For example, when you notice that you are irritable after an interaction with someone, spend a minute or so unpacking what happened and what specifically triggered you. After a while, this level of self-analysis will happen automatically. Alternatively, dedicate at least 10 minutes of your day to thinking about your shadow and the infinite ways it has manifested in your life.

Shadow Journaling

Shadow work journal prompts are a simple yet effective way to connect to your shadow regularly. The best part is that the questions have been prepared for you. All you need to do is schedule enough time to go through a few prompts during each session. Since journaling requires medium- to full-length responses, it is recommended to practice the technique in the evenings when you are relaxed and don't have any urgent tasks to attend to. Without the pressure of time, you can allow yourself to think about each prompt and provide rich and meaningful responses. The lists of journal prompts provided in this book are a great starting point. You can find many more themed journal prompts on the internet.

Inner Child Healing

Inner child healing is another popular form of therapy that is similar to shadow work. It seeks to connect you to your inner child, the aspect of your psyche that is rooted in your childhood, and heal unresolved issues and trauma that you never had the opportunity to address and recover from back then. Inner child healing can be done using the same techniques of shadow work like meditation, journaling, affirmations, and mirror work. However, the difference is that you are connecting and communicating with younger versions of yourself to listen and respond to their needs, fears, desires, and traumas. Inner child healing aims to reparent the child inside of you who didn't receive the love and security he or she needed and teach them healthier behaviors and coping mechanisms.

Humbling Yourself

A strong ego is normally associated with confidence. However, the truth is that a strong ego compensates for the lack of confidence and healthy self-esteem. When you possess genuine confidence and healthy self-esteem, you have a realistic and balanced perception of yourself. You are aware of your strengths and weaknesses and wholeheartedly accept both of them.

In contrast, when you lack confidence and have low self-esteem, you tend to overestimate your strengths and avoid confronting your weaknesses. To protect yourself from feeling inferior, you inflate your ego and develop a false sense of confidence known as arrogance. Arrogance distorts your sense of reality, which causes you to believe that you are superior to others (i.e., either mentally, emotionally, physically, or morally). This mentality makes it difficult for you to accept your undesirable traits, memories, or emotions.

The word *humble* comes from the root word *humility*, which refers to having a modest opinion of your importance. The process of shadow work requires humility because only then can you willingly explore dark traits that you would otherwise deny or hide. Humbling yourself brings you down to earth and causes you to pay attention to what you are thinking and feeling in every moment. It invites you to be honest and vulnerable about who you are and the good and bad experiences you have been through.

There are different ways to humble yourself. For instance, you can talk to people who come from different backgrounds and hear their life stories, volunteer at a shelter or support a social cause, practice empathy toward difficult people, or reflect on the hardship you have overcome over the years. All of this can be summarized as embracing the experience of being human and learning from both pleasant and unpleasant life situations.

Several years ago, author Minerva Siegel wrote a blog post sharing her journey practicing shadow work. At the time, she was looking for ways to improve her self-care routine and stumbled across this form of therapy. What enticed her was the ability of shadow work to uncover and release psychological deadweight that we all unconsciously carry to some extent. Minerva challenged herself to find shadow work practices that she resonated with and could easily be incorporated into her routine. In the end, she decided to go with journaling, creating shadow art, and paying attention to her inner dialogue.

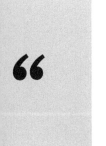

Regular journaling helped me realize I get a little self-destructive when I'm bored, and just that revelation about my shadow self was a huge step in the process of working on it. Now when I'm faced with boredom-induced impulses, I remember that self-destruction is a tendency I have and that I shouldn't indulge in these impulses while I'm in that bored headspace, as I may seriously regret them later. (Siegel, 2018)

About creating shadow art, she noted how the creative process encouraged her to express her feelings healthily and have some paintings to decorate her walls with. By paying attention to her inner dialogue, she could identify the voice of her inner critic and retrain herself to think positively.

Shadow work can be as simple, creative, and mentally stimulating as you choose to make it. The techniques provide a framework, which you can customize and make your own. You are more likely to enjoy shadow work when the practice becomes more than just therapy but rather a way of life. Therefore, take the time to consider how you desire to craft your shadow work journey.

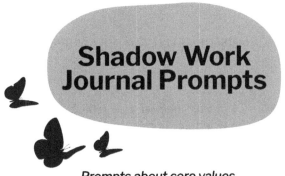

Shadow Work Journal Prompts

Prompts about core values

1. Reflect on a time when you strongly disagreed with someone's actions. Which of your values did they overlook? Why does this value matter to you?

2. Identify a past habit that you are ashamed to admit today. How did you develop this habit? What benefits did you receive from it? Why wouldn't it be acceptable today?

3. Do you have a relationship with someone who has different values
from you? How do you make the relationship work?
How do you manage projection when you are with them?

4. Describe a value that you care about but find difficult to express to others.
What thoughts or emotions get in the way of openly communicating this value?

5. Reflect on a time when you kept quiet about having one of your values undermined to avoid conflict in a relationship.
What can you learn from that experience?

Prompts about work

1. Are you satisfied with where you are currently in your career?
Make a list of concerns or grievances you have
and identify those within your control to act upon.

2. Take a moment to think about the fears holding you back from improving your work life. What are you unconsciously telling yourself? What past experiences have made you reluctant to go all in?

3. What career dreams were shattered or discouraged by your parents or caregivers as a child? How do you feel about those career dreams today?

**4. What social, cultural, or family expectations
have influenced your choice of work? Which of these expectations
clash with your beliefs and desires about work?**

**5. Describe your persona at work.
How is this persona similar and different from your persona at home?
How does this persona empower you and disempower you at the same time?**

Prompts about relationships

1. Describe what an ideal healthy relationship looks like to you. Identify a relationship in your life that comes close to this ideal and one that looks opposite to the ideal.

2. What are some of the toxic behaviors you tolerated from others in the past? What made you put up with those behaviors? Describe your psychological thought process and deeper issues this pattern revealed.

3. What is the one thing you needed from your parents that you didn't receive? How are you responding to that need today?

4. What are your assumptions about people of the opposite sex? Where do these assumptions come from? How have they influenced your relationships?

5. What emotional barriers prevent you from fully expressing your love to others?

Prompts about self-love

1. Describe your relationship with self-forgiveness. What are some things you find difficult to forgive yourself for? Why?

2. Empathize with your inner critic. How do they feel? What do they need?

3.In what ways do you self-sabotage? When do you usually do this? What is the motivation behind it?

4. How does it feel to be inside your body? What hurts? What feels good? What's missing? What do you have in abundance?

5. How important is it to be liked by others? How do you cope with rejection?

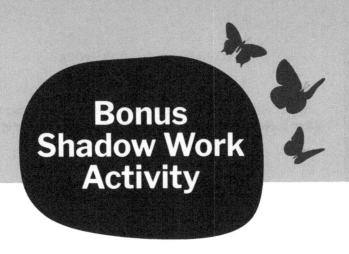

Create Your Mandala or Mandorla

The mandala and mandorla are creative shapes that are found in buildings and sacred temples, which carry both psychological and spiritual meaning. In shadow work, these shapes are drawn and colored to reflect the individual's state of mind and their path to wholeness.

The mandala is a geometric shape that is composed of many circles within circles. It symbolizes the relationship between self and creation. The colors used to decorate the mandala symbolize the harmony or disharmony within yourself or between yourself and others, or yourself and nature. You can also mix colors to illustrate a collision of two forces or states. When colors are mixed incorrectly, they create shades of grey or brown and represent dullness or monotony in your life. However, when blended correctly, they form a vibrant pattern and produce a rainbow mandala.

The mandorla is composed of two circles that meet to create a small almond shape in the middle. The meaning of a mandorla is the union or reconciliation of two opposing or contradicting natures. Think of your shadow self and conscious self. Whenever you draw a mandorla, pay attention to how small or large you create the center almond shape. The smaller the almond, the less integrated these two oppositional forces are. Metaphorically, the almond also represents your authentic self, the identity that is most balanced and grounded.

Each mandala you create will be a unique expression of how you feel at that particular time. While creating your shape, remain attuned to your mind and body. The following instructions will help you make a mandala from scratch using craft materials (Saxena, 2023):

1.   Place an 8.5" x 11" piece of paper on a flat surface.

2.   Take a ruler, find the center of the paper, and draw a small but visible dot.

3.   Using a sharp pencil and compass, draw circles around the dot in the center. The distance between your circles can be 0.5 or 1 inch.

4.   Pick up your ruler again and place it vertically on the page, in line with the center dot. Starting from the center, create rows of dots touching the periphery of each circle. Do this on both halves of the circle, as well as horizontally (the dots should make a "+" shape across the circle).

5.   Connect your dots with vertical and horizontal lines.

6.   Repeat the process and add more rows of dots going diagonally (the dots should make an "x" shape across the circle. Connect the dots with diagonal lines.

7.   At this stage, you have created the basic mandala framework. It is time to bring out your craft materials and draw repetitive shapes and symbols in each circle. Remember, what you draw on one half of the circle, you must mirror the other half too to create a harmonious mandala design.

Alternatively, use free templates online or mandala coloring books to color in your mandala. For your mandorla, feel free to draw it by hand (you can also add words inside the three connected shapes to represent what thoughts and emotions exist on both sides and in the middle).

You have learned about the ins and outs of shadow work, including what to avoid, and how to enhance your practice. The only thing left to do is to get started by incorporating one shadow work practice into your daily routine and celebrate the first of many milestones!

Spreading the Light

Now that you've equipped yourself with all the tools to embrace your hidden self and transcend emotional triggers and past traumas, it's time to share your newfound wisdom and guide others on their journey.

By simply sharing your honest opinion about this book on Amazon, you're not only helping fellow seekers find the guidance they need but also igniting their passion for shadow work.

Your contribution is invaluable. The essence of shadow work thrives when we pass on our knowledge, and you're playing a crucial role in keeping this transformative practice alive.

Thank you for your generosity. Together, we continue to light the way for those seeking self-discovery and personal growth, ensuring that the flame of shadow work never dims.

Scan the QR code to leave your review:

With Gratitude,
Lulu Nicholson.

PS - Did you know? Sharing something of value with another person enriches both of your lives. If you believe this book could illuminate someone else's path, consider passing it along.

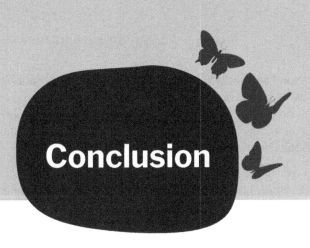

Conclusion

Shadow work is the way to illumination. When we become aware of all that is buried within us, that which is lurking beneath the surface no longer has power over us. –Aletheia Luna

Embark on the Journey of Becoming

Shadow work goes against your natural human instincts. Whenever you sense a potential threat, your default response is to become defensive, withdraw, or numb the sensation. This is what you have always done since you were a child, and it is an unconscious pattern that isn't easy to deconstruct and change.

Nevertheless, there come moments in life when facing your fears is the best thing to do. From a psychological standpoint, this means building the courage to confront past trauma, emotional issues, and destructive habits that have interfered with your quality of life. You will know when it is time to face your fears because the pain of denying your past becomes heavier than the pain of surrendering to the healing process.

Shadow work is not for everybody. It is specifically designed for those individuals who admit to being imperfect and are open to embracing and learning from their imperfections. The process of shadow work is intense and demands complete honesty in recognizing, exposing, naming, expressing, and accepting your undesirable traits and behaviors, as well as positive traits and behaviors that have been denied or shoved to the side.

This book has revealed both the benefits and implications of practicing shadow work and provided you with an in-depth look into the framework and techniques for getting the best results from this therapy. The book was broken down into three parts so you could understand the layers of the shadow work journey.

Part 1 offered an introduction to the concept of the shadow and basic guidelines on how to prepare for the process and navigate the roller coaster of emotions that may emerge. Building on this knowledge, Part 2 of the book explained how shadow work can be used to pull up and process unresolved trauma and challenge trauma-based reactions and behaviors. It also explored shadow integration, the practice of bringing up aspects of your shadow to the surface and integrating them into your conscious identity. Part 3 came full circle and focused on the positive ripple effects of shadow work, namely how the practice can enhance your relationships and help you build the life of your dreams, one exercise at a time.

You are not fully and wholeheartedly yourself until you have confronted your dark side and found meaning in the pain and suffering you have endured. Shadow work is a lifelong journey that continuously pushes you outside of your comfort zone to challenge and heal from the past, embrace the present moment, and become your authentic self. Commit today to incorporate shadow work into your daily routine and don't make any more excuses for not living your best life!

References

Abramson, A. (2021, November 1). *Cultivating empathy*. American Psychological Association. https://www.apa.org/monitor/2021/11/feature-cultivating-empathy

Academy of Ideas. (2020, February 27). *How to integrate your shadow – the dark side is unrealized potential*. Academy of Ideas. https://academyofideas.com/2020/02/how-to-integrate-your-shadow/

Aitchison, S. (2017, January 9). *5 powerful ways to work through fear*. Steven Aitchison. https://www.stevenaitchison.co.uk/5-powerful-ways-work-fear

Aletheia. (2022, November 16). *How to practice mirror work (six-step guide)*. LonerWolf. https://lonerwolf.com/mirror-work-guide/

American Association of Sensory Electrodiagnostic Medicine. (2023, May 28). *The truth hurts: Facing uncomfortable realities in life*. https://aasem.org/the-truth-hurts-facing-uncomfortable-realities-in-life/

Amercian Psychological Association. (2021). *Crisis hotlines and resources*. https://www.apa.org/topics/crisis-hotlines

Anderson, O. (2022, July 26). *35 shadow work quotes to help you accept and embrace your shadow self*. Mindful Zen. https://mindfulzen.co/shadow-work-quotes/

Asylab, C. (2023, November 27). *How "shadow work" has helped me in my mental health recovery*. The Mighty. https://themighty.com/topic/mental-health/shadow-work-help-mental-health/

Bismark, R. (2018, August 1). *Meditation shadow work: Dealing with darkness*. Yoga Medicine. https://yogamedicine.com/meditation-shadow-work-darkness/

Blain, T. (2023, May 11). *How does mindful communication impact mental health?* Verywell Mind. https://www.verywellmind.com/mindful-communication-definition-principles-benefits-how-to-do-it-7489103

Brown, L. (2020, July 14). *Shadow work: The complete guide to knowing your true self*. Idea Pod. https://ideapod.com/shadow-work/

Caspari, J. (2023, May 7). *Embracing vulnerability*. Psychology Today. https://www.psychologytoday.com/us/blog/living-well-when-your-body-doesnt-cooperate/202305/embracing-vulnerability

Chan, K. (2023, August 28). *Shadow work journal prompts: 50 prompts for your next session.* Psychedelic Support. https://psychedelic.support/resources/50-shadow-work-journal-prompts/

Chatt, K. (2022, December 26). *Intuitive art exercises to connect with your inner artist.* The Art and Beyond. https://theartandbeyond.com/intuitive-art-exercises/

Chesak, J. (2023, October 10). *Shadow work: Can TikTok's self-care trend improve your mental health?* Healthline. https://www.healthline.com/health-news/how-the-shadow-work-tiktok-trend-can-help-your-mental-health

Chira, M. (2023a, May 13). *Is shadow work dangerous? A comprehensive look at the pros and cons.* The Smart Read. https://www.thesmartread.com/post/is-shadow-work-dangerous

Chira, M. (2023b, May 13). *What is shadow work journaling? A comprehensive guide.* The Smart Read. https://www.thesmartread.com/post/what-is-shadow-work-journaling

Civico, A. (2014, April 21). *How self-awareness leads to effective communication.* Psychology Today. https://www.psychologytoday.com/us/blog/turning-point/201404/how-self-awareness-leads-effective-communication

Clarke, J. (2021, October 7). *Boost confidence and connections by celebrating success the right way.* Verywell Mind. https://www.verywellmind.com/healthy-ways-to-celebrate-success-4163887

Cleveland Clinic. (2023a, January 16). *Types of trauma and how to heal.* https://health.clevelandclinic.org/how-to-heal-from-trauma/

Cleveland Clinic. (2023b, August 1). *Tap into your dark side with shadow work.* Cleveland Clinic. https://health.clevelandclinic.org/shadow-work/

Cotec, I. (2021a, October 15). *Shadow work in relationship: Deeper intimacy in partnership.* HeroRise. https://www.herorise.us/shadow-work-in-relationship/

Cotec, I. (2021b, December 1). *Shadow work guided meditation: Integrating your shadow.* HeroRise. https://www.herorise.us/shadow-work-guided-meditation/#google_vignette

Davies, J. (2020, July 7). *Shadow work: 5 ways to use Carl Jung's technique to heal.* Learning Mind. https://www.learning-mind.com/shadow-work/

Dominica. (2022, December 27). *7 important reasons to bring shadow work into your mental health routine this year*. Daily Motivation. https://www.dailymotivation.site/7-important-reasons-to-bring-shadow-work-into-your-mental-health-routine-this-year/

Farah, S. (2015, February 4). *The archetypes of the anima and animus*. Applied Jung. https://appliedjung.com/the-archetypes-of-the-anima-and-animus/

Five healthy coping skills for facing setbacks. (2023, December 8). BetterHelp. https://www.betterhelp.com/advice/mindfulness/five-healthy-coping-skills-for-facing-setbacks/

Ford, D. (2022, July 26). *35 shadow work quotes to help you accept and embrace your shadow self*. Mindful Zen. https://mindfulzen.co/shadow-work-quotes/

Fritscher, L. (2023, November 20). *Overcoming a fear of vulnerability and love your imperfections*. Verywell Mind. https://www.verywellmind.com/fear-of-vulnerability-2671820

Gatt, R. (2023, June 3). *Identifying your trauma*. Woven Together Trauma Therapy. https://woventraumatherapy.com/blog/identify-your-trauma

Gilbert, A. (2022, April 7). *Is shadow work dangerous? Here's why some think so*. Soberish. https://www.soberish.co/is-shadow-work-dangerous/

Gillespie, B. (n.d.). *Self-compassion break script from Bob Gillespie*. https://www.fammed.wisc.edu/files/webfm-uploads/documents/research/stream/sc-break-script.pdf

Gillette, H. (2022a, March 29). *7 strategies to cope with emotional pain*. Psych Central. https://psychcentral.com/blog/how-to-deal-with-emotional-pain

Gillette, H. (2022b, April 4). *Can you become more empathetic? Absolutely, and here's how*. Psych Central. https://psychcentral.com/health/how-to-be-more-empathetic#how-to-act-empathetically

Gillihan, S. (2016, September 7). *21 common reactions to trauma*. Psychology Today. https://www.psychologytoday.com/us/blog/think-act-be/201609/21-common-reactions-trauma

Graham, S. (2022, July 26). *35 shadow work quotes to help you accept and embrace your shadow self*. Mindful Zen. https://mindfulzen.co/shadow-work-quotes/

Griffiths, N. (2021, September 15). *40 powerful affirmations for shadow work*. Seeking Serotonin. https://seekingserotonin.com/affirmations-for-shadow-work/?utm_content=cmp-true

Groves, O. (2022, January 21). *Shadow work journaling - what, why and how to do it*. Silk and Sonder. https://www.silkandsonder.com/blogs/news/shadow-work-journaling-what-why-how-to-do-it

Gupta, S. (2024, January 12). *What does it mean to feel overwhelmed?* Verywell Mind. https://www.verywellmind.com/feeling-overwhelmed-symptoms-causes-and-coping-5425548

Hall, A. (n.d.). *How to identify your shadow self: Discovering your hidden depths in 7 steps*. The Minds Journal. https://themindsjournal.com/how-to-identify-your-shadow-self/

Hanley-Dafoe, R. (2023, September 22). *5 ways to celebrate success and reaching your goals at work*. Psychology Today. https://www.psychologytoday.com/us/blog/everyday-resilience/202309/5-ways-to-celebrate-success-and-reaching-your-goals-at-work

The Happe World. (2023, April 13). *Benefits of shadow work and how to use it in your journey*. https://thehappeworld.com/benefits-of-shadow-work-and-how-to-use-it-in-your-journey/

Hardman, J. (2022, February 22). *How to do shadow work: A 4-step guide*. Josephine Hardman. https://josephinehardman.com/how-to-do-shadow-work-a-4-step-guide/

Hayes, S. C. (2023, November 16). *How to deal with your most overwhelming feelings*. Psychology Today. https://www.psychologytoday.com/us/blog/get-out-of-your-mind/202310/how-to-deal-with-overwhelming-feelings

Hetenyi, M. (2019, October 17). *Doing the shadow work to heal unprocessed pain and trauma*. Elephant Journal. https://www.elephantjournal.com/2019/10/shadow-work-is-metabolizing-grief/

Hill, L. (2023). Shadow work journal and workbook, updated edition: Discover your shadow self and heal from past trauma to find greater self-awareness, personal transformation and spiritual growth. https://www.amazon.com/Shadow-Work-Journal-Workbook-Updated/dp/B0CJLR22SD

Hill, T. (2015, June 3). *Facing our difficulties with the uncomfortable truth*. Tim Hill Psychotherapy. https://timhillpsychotherapy.com/when-the-truth-comes-roaring-in-1490/

Hogan, L. (2021, August 25). *How to be vulnerable*. WebMD. https://www.webmd.com/balance/features/how-to-be-vulnerable

Hussain, S. (2020, June 21). *Ken Wilber's 3-2-1 process: A method for retracting shadow projections*. Ox-Head Psychology. https://oxheadpsychology.com.au/ken-wilbers-3-2-1-process-a-method-for-retracting-shadow-projections/

Institute of Youth Development and Excellence. (2021, October 12). *How to recognize past trauma and its impact on your life*. https://iyde.org/blog/how-to-recognize-past-trauma-and-its-impact-on-your-life/

Irvine, M., & Meluch, R. (2020, March 2). *Not just a wife: celebrating the women behind famous men*. The DePaulia. https://depauliaonline.com/46963/artslife/not-just-a-wife-celebrating-the-women-behind-famous-men/

Jeffrey, S. (2017, January 2). *Psychological projection: How to reclaim the best parts of yourself*. Scott Jeffrey. https://scottjeffrey.com/psychological-projection/

Jeffrey, S. (2019, April 15). *Shadow work: A complete guide to getting to know your darker half*. Scott Jeffrey. https://scottjeffrey.com/shadow-work/

Johnson, R. A. (2013). *Owning your own shadow*. Harper Collins.

Jung, C. (2022, July 26). *35 shadow work quotes to help you accept and embrace your shadow self*. Mindful Zen. https://mindfulzen.co/shadow-work-quotes/

KamerPower. (2023, November 5). *What is shadow work meaning?: Benefits of shadow work*. KamerPower. https://kamerpower.com/what-is-shadow-work-meaning/

Kate, G. (2023, February 20). *45 journal prompts for shadow work (and what each one tells us)*. The Goal Chaser. https://thegoalchaser.com/journal-prompts-for-shadow-work/

King, K. (2019, April 30). *Understanding the long shadow of trauma*. Psychology Today. https://www.psychologytoday.com/us/blog/lifespan-perspectives/201904/understanding-the-long-shadow-trauma

Kirsten, C. (2023, March 7). *78 deep shadow work prompts to heal, grow and find yourself*. Typically Topical. https://typicallytopical.com/shadow-work-prompts/

Kunst, J. (2021, December 21). *Can you handle the truth?* Psychology Today. https://www.psychologytoday.com/us/blog/headshrinkers-guide-the-galaxy/201112/can-you-handle-the-truth

Kurland, B. (2022, August 22). *How to find comfort and ease amid difficult emotions.* Psychology Today. https://www.psychologytoday.com/us/blog/the-well-being-toolkit/202208/how-find-comfort-and-ease-amid-difficult-emotions

Lebow, H. I. (2023, January 21). *How does your body remember trauma? Plus 5 ways to heal.* Psych Central. https://psychcentral.com/health/how-your-body-remembers-trauma#how-to-heal-trauma

Leonard, J. (2020, June 3). *What is trauma? Types, symptoms, and treatments.* Medical News Today. https://www.medicalnewstoday.com/articles/trauma

Lewis, J. (2023, July 29). *Shadow self: what is it and how can it help you?* Zella Life. https://www.zellalife.com/blog/shadow-self-what-is-it-and-how-can-it-help-you/

Lim, S. (2020, April 8). *13 great ways how to celebrate small victories and make progress.* Stunning Motivation. https://stunningmotivation.com/celebrate-small-victories/

Lohret, K. (n.d.). *Understanding resistance and shadow.* Sage Hil Healing. https://www.sagehillhealing.com/understanding-resistance-and-shadow

Lucius. (2023, April 16). *Healing your relationships through shadow work: 30 shadow work prompts for relationships.* Shadow Work Journal. https://shadowworkjournal.com/shadow-work-prompts-for-relationships/

Luna, A. (n.d.). *Aletheia Luna quote.* Goodreads. https://www.goodreads.com/author/show/7360921.Aletheia_Luna

Lynch, E. (n.d.). *Evanna Lynch quote.* Goodreads. https://www.goodreads.com/author/show/7255387.Evanna_Lynch

Lynne, T. (n.d.). *Shadow integration.* The Courage Practice. https://thecouragepractice.org/shadowintegration

Main, P. (2023, March 30). *Carl Jung's archetypes.* Structural Learning. https://www.structural-learning.com/post/carl-jungs-archetypes

Maximus, D. (2022, July 26). *35 shadow work quotes to help you accept and embrace your shadow self.* Mindful Zen. https://mindfulzen.co/shadow-work-quotes/

Mayer, B. A. (2021, July 27). *Do you have a dark side? Shadow work experts say yes.* Healthline. https://www.healthline.com/health/mental-health/shadow-work#repression

Mental Health America. (n.d.). *Eighteen ways to cope with frustration.* https://www.mhanational.org/18-ways-cope-frustration

Moonster Leather Products. (2023, April 19). *Seven benefits of shadow journaling (and how to get started).* https://moonsterleather.com/blogs/news/shadow-journaling

Morin, A. (2023, November 3). *40 coping skills that will help you fight stress.* Verywell Mind. https://www.verywellmind.com/forty-healthy-coping-skills-4586742

Nash, J. (2023, September 26). *7 best breathwork techniques and exercises to use.* Positive Psychology. https://positivepsychology.com/breathwork-techniques/

Nicogossian, C. (2021, May 7). *What are shadow emotions? A psychologist explains how to identify yours.* Mindbodygreen. https://www.mindbodygreen.com/articles/shadow-emotions

Ono, Y. (2022, July 26). *35 shadow work quotes to help you accept and embrace your shadow self.* Mindful Zen. https://mindfulzen.co/shadow-work-quotes/

Othership. (2021, October 17). *Breathwork for healing trauma: 3 popular techniques and benefits.* https://www.othership.us/resources/breathwork-for-healing-trauma

Perry, E. (2022, June 13). *8 benefits of shadow work and how to start practicing it.* BetterUp. https://www.betterup.com/blog/shadow-work

Raypole, C. (2020, November 13). Emotional triggers: Defintion and how to manage them. *Healthline.* https://www.healthline.com/health/mental-health/emotional-triggers#finding-yours

Regan, S. (2021, November 11). *How to embrace and integrate your shadow self for major healing.* Mindbodygreen. https://www.mindbodygreen.com/articles/shadow-self

Resnick, A. (2022, February 3). *10 ways to heal from trauma.* Verywell Mind. https://www.verywellmind.com/10-ways-to-heal-from-trauma-5206940

Robinson, L., Segal, J., & Smith, M. (2023). *Effective communication.* Help Guide. https://www.helpguide.org/articles/relationships-communication/effective-communication.htm

Ryder, G. (2022, January 4). *What is trauma? Effects, causes, types, and how to heal.* Psych Central. https://psychcentral.com/health/what-is-trauma#related-conditions

Sasha. (2021, June 12). *70+ powerful shadow work prompts for deep reflection and growth.* Vital Ethos. https://www.vitalethos.com/shadow-work-prompts/

Saxena, A. (2023, October 22). *What is mandala and how to create mandala art.* LinkedIn. https://www.linkedin.com/pulse/what-mandala-how-create-art-arti-saxena/

Shadow integration 101. (2019, April 3). The Lovett Center. https://thelovettcenter.com/shadow-integration-101/

Sherman, A. (2021, January 10). *The 7 skills necessary to overcome fear.* Psychology Today. https://www.psychologytoday.com/intl/blog/dysfunction-interrupted/202101/the-7-skills-necessary-overcome-fear

Siegel, M. (2018, August 20). *Why I made working on my shadow self part of my self-care routine.* Elite Daily. https://www.elitedaily.com/p/your-shadow-self-meaning-should-be-a-crucial-part-of-your-self-care-heres-why-10159688

Spiritual Primate. (2023, May 23). *50 shadow work prompts for childhood trauma.* https://spiritualprimate.com/50-powerful-shadow-work-prompts-for-healing-childhood-trauma/

Substance Abuse and Mental Health Services Administration (US). (2014). *Understanding the impact of trauma.* National Library of Medicine. https://www.ncbi.nlm.nih.gov/books/NBK207191/

Swaim, E. (2022, May 25). *7 things to remember on your trauma recovery journey.* Healthline. https://www.healthline.com/health/mental-health/trauma-recovery#set-your-own-pace

Tiodar, A. (2023, May 22). *7 powerful shadow work techniques and practices.* Subconscious Servant. https://subconsciousservant.com/shadow-work-techniques/

Tulane University. (2020, December 8). *Understanding the effects of social isolation on mental health.* https://publichealth.tulane.edu/blog/effects-of-social-isolation-on-mental-health/

Tunstall, K. (2021, August 8). *35 powerful shadow work affirmations to help you heal and grow.* Refined Prose. https://www.refinedprose.com/shadow-work-affirmations/

Villines, Z. (2022, August 30). *What is shadow work? Benefits and exercises.* Medical News Today. https://www.medicalnewstoday.com/articles/what-is-shadow-work#in-spirituality

Williamson, J. (2019, July 23). *Ho'oponopono prayer for forgiveness, healing and making things right.* Healing Brave. https://healingbrave.com/blogs/all/hooponopono-prayer-for-forgiveness

Winch, G. (2014, July 2). *The secret to overcoming any setback.* Psychology Today. https://www.psychologytoday.com/us/blog/the-squeaky-wheel/201407/the-secret-to-overcoming-any-setback

Wooll, M. (2022, June 13). *8 benefits of shadow work and how to start practicing it.* BetterUp. https://www.betterup.com/blog/shadow-work

Wright, K. W. (2023, March 22). *Unlock the benefits of shadow work journaling.* Day One. https://dayoneapp.com/blog/shadow-work-journaling/